Depression

Anxiety

A Self Help Guide to Stop Worrying, Eliminate Anxiety, Remove Negative Thoughts and Recover From Phobias, Ptsd Using Nlp and Cbt

(How to Stop Overthinking and Live Your Life)

Daniel Huebner

Published by Kevin Dennis

© Daniel Huebner

All Rights Reserved

Depression Therapy: A Self Help Guide to Stop Worrying, Eliminate Anxiety, Remove Negative Thoughts and Recover From Phobias, Ptsd Using Nlp and Cbt (How to Stop Overthinking and Live Your Life)

ISBN 978-1-989920-85-5

All rights reserved. No part of this guide may be reproduced in any form without permission in writing from the publisher except in the case of brief quotations embodied in critical articles or reviews.

Legal & Disclaimer

The information contained in this book is not designed to replace or take the place of any form of medicine or professional medical advice. The information in this book has been provided for educational and entertainment purposes only.

The information contained in this book has been compiled from sources deemed reliable, and it is accurate to the best of the Author's knowledge; however, the Author cannot guarantee its accuracy and validity and cannot be held liable for any errors or omissions. Changes are periodically made to this book. You must consult your doctor or get professional medical advice before using any of the suggested remedies, techniques, or information in this book.

Upon using the information contained in this book, you agree to hold harmless the Author from and against any damages, costs, and expenses, including any legal fees potentially resulting from the application of any of the information provided by this guide. This disclaimer applies to any damages or injury caused by the use and application, whether directly or indirectly, of any advice or information presented, whether for breach of contract, tort, negligence, personal injury, criminal intent, or under any other cause of action.

You agree to accept all risks of using the information presented inside this book. You need to consult a professional medical practitioner in order to ensure you are both able and healthy enough to participate in this program.

TABLE OF CONTENTS

INTRODUCTION 1

CHAPTER 1: SOCIAL ACTIVITY 6

CHAPTER 2: TYPES OF ANXIETY DISORDERS IN CHILDREN AND ADULTS 10

CHAPTER 3: UNDERSTANDING BIPOLAR DISORDER 17

CHAPTER 4: DIFFERENCE AND SIMILARITIES BETWEEN ANXIETY AND FEAR 27

CHAPTER 5: SELF MANAGEMENT TO STOP STRESS 37

CHAPTER 6: DEPRESSION: THE BASICS 42

CHAPTER 7: DISCOVERY OF THOUGHT FIELD THERAPY AND EMOTIONAL FREEDOM TECHNIQUE 50

CHAPTER 8: WHAT IS STRESS? 56

CHAPTER 9: UNDERSTANDING DEPRESSION..................... 60

CHAPTER 10: ALL YOU NEED TO KNOW ABOUT SOCIAL ANXIETY AND SOCIAL PHOBIA... 64

CHAPTER 11: HOW CAN TAPPING BENEFIT YOU? 71

CHAPTER 12: HOW CAN AROMATHERAPY HELP TO REDUCE ANXIETY? 75

CHAPTER 13: WHAT IS ANXIETY? 77

CHAPTER 14: THE F-E-A-R-L-E-S-S MANTRA 79

CHAPTER 15: PRINCIPLES OF MEDITATION 87

CHAPTER 16: THERAPY FOR PANIC ATTACKS AND ANXIETY 91

CHAPTER 17: REALIZE, ACCEPT AND MANAGE................ 96

CHAPTER 18: GROUP THERAPY..................................... 102

CHAPTER 19: TURNING RELAXATION TECHNIQUES INTO HABITS 105

CHAPTER 20: FEARS AND DEPRESSION ASSOCIATED WITH NARCISSISTIC ABUSE 111

CHAPTER 21: WHY AND HOW TO FOCUS ON OTHERS ... 118

CHAPTER 22: TACKLING ANXIETY 126

CHAPTER 23: SPEAK YOUR MIND................................... 141

CHAPTER 24: HARD TRAUMA AND SOFT TRAUMA 147

CHAPTER 25: YOU HAVE THE POWER 155

CHAPTER 26: SUPPLEMENTS.. 163

CHAPTER 27: THE ULTIMATE CHEAT SHEET ON INTROVERTS AT WORK.. 170

CHAPTER 28: MIND-READING AND ASSUMING 174

CHAPTER 29: UNDERSTANDING WHERE YOUR SHYNESS AND ANXIETIES ARE COMING FROM 180

CHAPTER 30: TODAY IS A NEW DAY 185

CHAPTER 31: CLONAZEPAM PRONOUNCED AS (KLOE NA' ZE PAM) 194

CONCLUSION 201

INTRODUCTION

Who does not feel anxious at times? Everyone feels anxious sometimes.

Typical situations that cause individuals to feel anxious could be preparing for exams, going to job interviews, or meeting deadlines for projects at work. Some anxiety is part of human nature. It can help people prepare for an unknown future. It also propels them to develop plans to cope with future challenges. As brothers Chip and Dan Heath (2010) explained, the emotional side of our brain can drive us to act and complete tasks. Anxiety is one of several emotions that triggers us to get things done daily.

Why am I talking about anxiety? Anxiety can cause severe health problems if it becomes excessive. This can impact every aspect of people's lives: work, family, relationships and recreation. People who experience intense fear and worry may be suffering from an anxiety disorder. Anxiety can be debilitating, especially when a person is dealing with multiple stressors in life. They may feel overwhelmed by anxious feelings and physical symptoms almost every day. Anxiety is experienced throughout the body. For example, you may feel changes in your heartbeat, some pressure in the chest and some difficulty breathing.

As a psychologist, I have worked with youth and adults in my practice over the past decade. I've noticed more teenage girls and young women complain of anxiety each year. It appears young women were more likely to have anxiety during recent years. The anxiety epidemic was reported on in many research studies and the national news during 2016 and 2017. Recent studies report anxiety has increased among teens and young women of the "Gen Z" and "Millennial" generations.

The good news is, anxiety disorders are treatable, and many treatment options are available. I have seen many patients recover from anxiety disorders. The intensity of anxiety often went down to 1 or 2 on a scale of 0-10. Recognizing, understanding and treating anxiety among girls and women is critical.

I've written this book in the hope that this information will help readers learn to recognize and understand when their loved ones and friends are suffering from anxiety disorders and support them. Parents can prevent their children from developing anxiety disorders if they recognize, understand and treat it in an early stage. If your child has excessive anxiety, you can help him or her to cope with it via psychotherapy and other ways.

In this book, I focus on anxiety among teenage girls ("Gen Z") and young women ("Millennial girls"). In Chapter One, normal anxiety and abnormal anxiety are discussed and defined. Anxiety disorders are explained based on the Diagnostic Statistical Manual.

In Chapter Two, the potential causes of anxiety disorders are discussed. Biological explanation refers to genetic transmissions of anxiety from parents to their children. Environmental explanation includes parenting as well as mobile phone and internet use. Life transitions and developmental issues for girls and women are categorized into the five stages from childhood to adulthood. I intend to highlight developmental tasks and possible stressors that may trigger their anxiety.

In Chapter Three, the "anxiety epidemic" is explained based on recent reports. Anxiety among girls has recently significantly increased. This upsurge appears to be connected to the prevalence of mobile phone use and social media obsession.

In Chapter Four, evidence-based treatments for anxiety disorders, including cognitive-behavioral therapy and medications are explained. In addition, alternative, holistic, and body-mind approaches such as sleep, nutrition, exercise and family and peer support are explored and discussed.

In Chapter Five, emotional intelligence and self-compassion are explored for prevention of anxiety disorders among girls. These psychological concepts can be incorporated into future treatments of anxiety disorders.

Helpful resources related to anxiety and mental health are provided at the back of the book, along with a complete list of references and an Appendix.

Chapter 1: Social Activity

As mentioned above, social activity can be the panacea that we need to try and combat anxiety. Anxiety can become a deeply dangerous feeling, and trying to come at it alone is not good for the mind. Dealing with all of your problems alone is a massive burden on the body as much as the soul.

It can compress how we feel about ourselves, our talents and how likely we are to find a solution to our issues. The only issue is that, like many people, you probably feel like you are alone.

I know I did. When I did know people wanted to help, I felt like my problems were simply not theirs to contend with. "Why would they care?" was my go-to way of thinking when feeling anxious. I didn't want to burden people with my problems, and thought I was being a hero for being so thoughtful.

Really, I was being extremely selfish. Not reaching out to the people in your life who care is going to halt you from making any kind of progress. We feel like others will not understand how we feel, but they don't need to fully understand.

They just need to know.

Anxiety can make us crude, rude and hard to be around at the best of times. It creates a reactionary, negative mindset in many people that can become very challenging to be around. This comes from the fact we think others won't be able to "get" the issues that we are facing.

Feeling this way can create the kind of mindset that stops us from making any kind of long-term progress in life, and halts us from making a distinctive step forward with our anxiety. Here are some things to try and keep in mind when it comes to the social aspect:

- There's no shame in admitting you feel this way. 18% of adults suffer from the affliction – the chances are that you are not alone. You aren't the lone wolf here, or the odd one out. Nobody thinks you are being dramatic, or over the top, about how you feel.

- Reaching out really does help. Whether it's a family member, a friend or even a professional from a support group, talking helps. It lets you see your own situation in a clearer way and, crucially, it can help you see that many of the things you feel anxious over have yet to happen, or may never happen.
- Human contact can help the healing process accelerate. A simple holding of the hand, a hug or even a handshake can reinforce our self-belief and inner confidence.
- Remember, you are more than JUST an anxious person. You have talents, skills, attributes and achievements. When people remind you of this, listen to them. They aren't saying it to be nice or to "pep you up" – people can spot your positive

attributes far better than your anxious mind can.

- The social impact on your anxiety can be hard to deal with, if you don't let your mind take in what others are telling you. You'll become more shut off and harder to be around in time. When people extend the hand of friendship or family, don't reject it.

You might be feeling awful inside, but friendship and human affection can help just that.

Chapter 2: Types Of Anxiety Disorders In Children And Adults

Anxiety attacks can affect people of all ages, including children. In fact, anxiety disorders are the most common type of mental health disorder in children, affecting as many as one in ten of young people. Anxiety and panic attacks in children is more common than you would think.

What causes anxiety in children?

There are many factors that cause children to develop anxiety problems, two of which are genetic and environmental factors. During their lives all children experience some kind of anxiety, this is normal and to be expected.

For example, when children start school for the first time they worry about being left without their parents for the first time, and most children are scared of the dark so they become distressed. Such anxiety becomes a problem when it interrupts a child's normal activities like attending school and making friends or sleeping.

Anxiety can affect a child's ability to function properly, and they may develop high blood pressure, start to vomit, and experience stomach pains among other things.

Types of anxiety disorders in children and adults.

Generalized anxiety disorder or GAD.

Children and adults with generalized anxiety disorder experience fears and worries that they find difficult to control. They worry about almost everything - school, home life, sports, and being on time etc.

They may be restless, irritable tense or easily tired, and they may have trouble concentrating or sleeping. Children with GAD are usually eager to please others and look for perfection in everything they do.

Children with separation anxiety disorder

Children with separation anxiety disorder are so worried about being away from home it affects their ability to function socially and at school. Children with this problem need to stay home near to their parents.

Children with this disorder may worry excessively about their parents when they are apart from them. When they are together, the child may cling to parents, refuse to go to school, or be afraid to sleep alone. Repeated nightmares about separation and physical symptoms such as stomach-aches and headaches are also common in children with separation anxiety disorder.

Post-traumatic stress disorder (PTSD)

Children who experience a physical or emotional trauma such as witnessing a shooting or disaster, surviving physical, emotional or sexual abuse, or being in a car accident may develop post-traumatic stress disorder (PTSD). Children are more easily traumatized than adults.

An event that may not be traumatic to an adult - such as a bumpy plane journey - might be traumatic to a child. A child may "re-experience" the trauma through nightmares, constant thoughts about what happened, or re-enacting the event while playing.

A child with PTSD will experience symptoms of general anxiety, including irritability or trouble sleeping and eating. Children may exhibit other symptoms such as being easily startled.

Social phobia

Social phobia usually emerges in the mid-teens. Young people with this disorder have a constant fear of social situations or when they have to perform such as speaking in class or eating in public. The fear is often accompanied by physical symptoms such as sweating, blushing, heart palpitations, shortness of breath, or muscle tenseness.

Young people with social phobia typically respond to these feelings by avoiding the feared situation. For example, they may stay home from school or avoid parties. Young people with social phobia are often overly sensitive to criticism, have trouble being assertive, and suffer from low self-esteem.

Social phobia can be limited to specific situations, so the adolescent may fear dating and avoid recreational events but can still be confident in academic and work situations.

Obsessive-compulsive disorder (OCD)

Obsessive-compulsive disorder typically begins in early childhood or adolescence. Children can show symptoms at a very young age and may have frequent and uncontrollable thoughts and may perform routines or rituals in an attempt to eliminate the thoughts. Those with the disorder often repeat behaviors to avoid some imagined consequence.

For example, a compulsion common to people with OCD is excessive hand washing due to fear of germs. Other common compulsions include counting, repeating works silently, and rechecking completed tasks. These obsessions and compulsions take up so much time that they interfere with daily living and cause a young person a great deal of anxiety.

Panic disorder - panic attacks - children

Children and adolescents with panic disorder have unexpected and repeated periods of intense fear or discomfort along with other symptoms such as racing heartbeat or feeling short of breath. These panic attacks can last from minutes to hours.

Panic disorder often begins during adolescence, although it may start during childhood. Panic attacks can interfere with a child's or adolescent's relationships, schoolwork and, and normal development. Children and adolescents with panic disorder may begin to feel anxious most of the time, even when they are not having a panic attack.

Some children with panic disorder develop depression and may be at risk of suicidal behavior. As an attempt to decrease anxiety, some adolescents with panic disorder will use alcohol or drugs.

Chapter 3: Understanding Bipolar Disorder

Having mood swings is natural; everyone has experienced times when they are happy one minute then completely depressed the next. Now imagine having an average mood swing and then multiply it by several times - that is what it feels like to have bipolar disorder. Sometimes these erratic mood swings can be so severe that it can affect the sufferer's career and personal relationships, and there are even some who have committed suicide because their minds can no longer handle the stress it is experiencing.

If you feel like your emotions are getting out of control lately, and you are starting to experience negative things because of them, then you might have bipolar disorder yourself. You need to understand as much as you can about this ailment so you can get the necessary medical assistance before it gets any worse.

What is Bipolar Disorder?

Bipolar disorder is a condition of the brain which causes recurring episodes where the person's moods will switch from a high-energy, manic state to an almost debilitating depression. These moods are so far from each other that they are considered polar opposites, hence the name "bipolar." These extreme manic-depressive episodes usually lasts for a couple of days or weeks at a time (with normal periods in between them), but in several extreme cases, the episodes can last for months and often results in serious health degradation.

Unlike other mental health issues, it is only recently that people have become aware of bipolar disorder, which is why around 70% of people who actually have this ailment do not get an accurate diagnosis; most of the time bipolar disorder is mistaken for depression, and this actually makes things worse for the sufferer.

Among the people who develop bipolar disorder, most usually experience a depression before they experience their manic state, and some only experience hypomania, which is a less severe manic episode. Two out of three people who experience the depressive state first tend to seek help in dealing with their problem, compare that with the people who experience the manic state first wherein almost all will not even recognize that they have a problem at all. If you think you are at risk of developing bipolar disorder it is best that you get screened and monitored for the condition so that you can do something about it before it becomes unmanageable.

The Different Types of Bipolar Disorder

What makes diagnosing bipolar disorder a bit tricky is the fact that there are three kinds that you need to watch out for.

Bipolar I - This is the classic case of the disorder, in fact, most people think that this is the only type of bipolar disorder there is. This type of disorder is characterized by having at least one manic or mixed episode and usually one depressive state.

Bipolar II - In this case, the person affected does not experience the type of full-blown manic episodes like the ones in Bipolar I. With this type of bipolar disorder, the sufferer goes through episodes of hypomania (mild manic states) and severe bouts of depression. This is the type of bipolar disorder that is usually misdiagnosed as depression because the sufferer does not really notice his/her manic episodes.

Cyclothymia - This is a mild form of bipolar disorder where the person only experiences cyclical bouts of hypomania and mild depression. Most of the time, people who have cyclothymia do not even seek help because their symptoms are significantly less severe than full-blown bipolar disorder, they are so mild in fact, that they do not really affect their quality of life at all.

Causes and Triggers that Cause Bipolar Disorder in People

There is no singular cause of bipolar disorder, and this makes it harder to catch the ailment before it gets worse. There are some people who are genetically predisposed to have bipolar disorder, and yet they do not even develop a mild case of it; this means that besides a person's genetics, there must be other factors that can cause bipolar disorder in people. Researches show that abnormal thyroid functions, a faulty biological clock, and hormone imbalances can also make a person more prone to developing manic-depressive episodes.

And then there are external and psychological factors, or "triggers", that cause the development of bipolar disorder in people, namely:

Excessive amounts of stress - If a person is genetically predisposed to developing bipolar disorder, huge amounts of stress can and will make sure that it happens. It has been observed that in most cases, the stresses involved in life-changing events like getting married, moving away from home, or the death of a loved one can trigger manic or depressive episodes in people.

Substance abuse - Although studies made on the connection of substance abuse and bipolar disorders have been inconclusive, they have been proven to make existing conditions worse. For instance, cocaine, ecstasy, and other amphetamines have been observed to make a person's manic episodes much more extreme, while depressants like alcohol and tranquilizers can make depressive episodes worse.

Sleep deprivation - It was mentioned earlier that sudden changes in a person's biological clock can trigger the onset of bipolar disorder, and nothing messes up your circadian rhythm more than not getting enough sleep at night.

Medication - Certain prescription drugs, namely antidepressants, can also trigger bipolar manic episodes. Substances like caffeine, thyroid medications, appetite suppressants, and other types of medications can actually make a sufferer's manic states last longer and feel more intense.

Changes in the seasons - Seasonal changes have also been observed to cause manic/depressive episodes in people prone to bipolar disorders. Spring and summer seems to trigger manic states, while the colder parts of the year are said to cause depressive states.

Common Myths and Misconceptions About Bipolar Disorder

People with bipolar disorder switch back and forth between manic and depressive states - Although this is the characteristic of having bipolar disorder, the mood swings are often not like what most people assume them to be. Some sufferers experience depression more often and longer than manias; in some people, the manic states are so mild that they sometimes fail to notice them when they come.

Besides affecting the person's moods, bipolar disorder does not really have any other ill effects on a person - A lot of people take bipolar disorder lightly, what they do not know is that it is more than just having mood swings. People who have bipolar disorder often have low energy levels, reduced sex drives, find it hard to concentrate and make wise decisions, and this even causes most people to turn to substance abuse just so they can cope with what they are feeling. Other researches also suggest that there is a connection between bipolar disorders and the development of chronic ailments like heart disease, diabetes, and others.

Besides taking medication, there is nothing else you can do to treat bipolar disorder -

Yes, it is true that it is almost impossible to keep bipolar disorder in check without the use of certain types of medication, but that does not mean that it is the only way you can treat it. You can drastically minimize the effects of your manic/depressive episodes by exercising, eating healthy, and avoiding things that cause you stress.

It is impossible for people with bipolar disorder to lead normal, healthy lives - Nothing is impossible, even if you have bipolar disorder, it is possible for you to live a regular, and happy life with the help of proper coping techniques and treatments. If you are diagnosed with bipolar disorder, do not feel like it is the end of the world, there is still hope.

Knowing more about this mental condition is the first step towards recovery. If you have even the slightest inkling that you may have bipolar disorder then it is about time that you seek help, or at least try to treat yourself before your condition becomes too much for you to handle.

Chapter 4: Difference And Similarities

Between Anxiety And Fear

Well, you might make some clear distinction between anxiety and fear, but most people cannot. Sometimes, it's just a way of saying one thing in two different words. Recall someone saying they are fearful of heights. The same people may say they are anxious of heights. Basically, they are confused about their own feelings.

Our body responds differently to both these situations. There are different nerves in our body which get active when we feel fear or anxiety. For instance, if an intruder points a gun on your temple, you will definitely have fearful feelings. These feelings are completely different from dizziness, mild nausea or butterflies in the stomach if you are going for an interview. The latter can be termed as anxiety.

Anxiety is also used to describe situations when you have a chronic feeling of tension or worry, the basis of which is not clear. There are much more differences between fear and anxiety. You can have short term response of fear when you see a cockroach in your bedroom. But, if you are anxious about something, you may get up at two in the morning and cannot sleep again.

By whatever name you call your feelings of restlessness, your main focus should be on the fact that how you prepare yourself to tackle such situations. You need to look in the eyes of these uninvited guests with patience and you will be able to figure out their mischief. You do not have to allow them to have a firm grip on your life.

Anxiety and Fear in Detail

Imagine an anxiety scale, which has mild concern and worry on one end. The scale progresses through fear and anxiety. On the other end, there are blind panic and fear. Let us understand the differences more clearly.

Anxiety and Worry: These reactions come under the set of response, which you give to an ill-defined or imprecise threat. You just anticipate them in advance and create the fear in your mind. These feelings can be associated with the requirement to be gear up. Worrying for something leads the way to anxiety.

Panic and Fear: These responses come under the set of reactions, which you give to a well-defined threat. These threats come can be vividly imagined or real. These feelings are mainly associated with escape and avoidance. Panic is the extreme form of fear.

Worry

This process of thinking gives birth to emotions and feelings articulated as anxiety. Sometimes, worrying can be useful in finding answers to problems. But, if you worry too much about the problems which do not have an immediate solution, you may become pessimistic and laden with negative feelings of unseen troubles.

This way, you are misusing your imagination. Worrying too much can generate conditions which make you anxious, such as

Helplessness: You do not have sufficient information to tackle the difficult situations.

Incongruity: Different pieces of information, conflicting to each other.

Over Stimulation: Information overload or excess of information.

Unpredictability: You are not sure about the outcome.

Anxiety

The feeling of anxiety is more like a warning. It gives you a yellow alert when you are anxious about something. People often try to find out surety in unsure situations. They try to stay alert and safe of possible dangers. They use anxiousness as a tactic to survive- by trying to plan in advance for every possible hazard. Sometimes, you might have also worried about future. But, future is unpredictable and thus the outcomes of your present actions cannot be easily determined today. That is why; you have so many "what if" situations in your life at such times.

When you are excessively anxious, your body undergoes the following changes:

Heightened Senses: You start looking for dangers everywhere.

Jumpiness: Your mind always feels on the edge of falling.

Tensed Muscles: Your muscles tense up if any kind of physical action is needed in case of anxiety.

The approach of anxiousness serves us well when we have to confront a genuine potential hazard. For instance, when the soldiers are wandering in the forests, they have to be anxious about potential threats from animals. Whenever they hear a hustle from the bushes, they turn around immediately with their weapons to look for enemy and harmful animals. If it comes out to be just a blast of air, there is nothing to lose. However, it is not really helpful if you keep evaluating a situation of future in your mind day and night.

When you forecast scenarios of disaster, it leads to feelings of fear and apprehension. Even if the disasters have the least possibilities of happening, you begin to imagine what the situation would be like if the disasters take place. It is important to note that our mind cannot distinguish between imagination and reality. Thus, it starts experiencing fear.

Fear

You have already read that fear is linked with dangers that are certain and you need to figure out tactics of survival like flight or fight. Fear can be termed as "orange alert", which is one step higher than anxiety but one step lower than panic. This can also be based on something imaginary or real. The amount of fear is dependent on:

The unpleasantness or seriousness of threat

The proximity of the event to the present

When you are fearful of something in anticipation, you are only worried about the future. It has nothing to do with the present. Had it been linked with the present, you would have been taking action, not thinking about it. The future event is not yet classified as a threat to your life. That is why; you have not yet reached the level of panic. However, your body starts to engage in the response of flight or fight, particularly when you are intensely imagining the situation. Your body may undergo the following changes:

Rapid Breathing: You start taking in more oxygen than normal.

Sweating: It happens naturally to give a better grip to your hands as well as cool down your body.

Raised Heartbeat: It happens so that your heart may pump more blood rich in oxygen to the muscles which have already received a high dose of adrenalin.

Sometimes, you may be in the state of fear for longer periods than normal, when your thoughts are not in your control. You may even feel extremely tired after you have felt anxious or fearful for a long time even if you were sitting idle. Fear should be aimed at survival in the short term, not the existence for long term.

Panic

Panic is the extreme form of fear. When you are under the state of panic, you feel overwhelmed by the mental and physical feelings of your mind. The present conditions of danger make you panic. Such dangers may be life threatening. Panic may be termed as "red alert". It may get your body into the best possible position of survival. You prepare your body for flight or fight. You might even freeze sometimes if your mind is not able to think beyond a limit.

You might have heard of panic attacks. It implies a sudden rush of overpowering fear. Your heart starts pounding and you are not able to breathe. You might even feel like dying or going mad. This is more than the red alert. It must be treated immediately after diagnosis. It may lead to other panic disorders. People are often withdrawn from other normal activities of their lives. However, it is possible to cure panic attacks and reduce the symptoms to gain control over your life again. It is only when you realize that the panic attack has strikes for no obvious reason, when you become aware of the physical changes in your body.

Depression

Though you might think that depression is not related to any of the above situations, but the fact is that many people go into depression due to fear, anxiety, worry, and panic. Depression, many a times, accompanies the above stated conditions. However, it is not directly related to such situations, depression does share many negative thoughts you experience otherwise. If you are under the condition of chronic anxiety or fear, which leave you feeling overwhelmed, you may start feeling that your life is hopeless, which is the prominent trait of depression.

Chapter 5: Self Management To Stop Stress

Too little time, boss pushing for work to be finished, kids are annoying you, bills to pay, store shopping to be done, house work to do, partner requesting your help... Can this seem like a familiar circumstance in your life? Stress is usually with us managing what we do and how we feel. If you're pressured you do things quicker and in an unhappier way. You either become aggressive towards other individuals as a form of releasing the stress or you grow to be submissive by hiding the stress.

When you are submissive and hiding your stress, it internally eats at you hurting your inner thoughts and your relationships. When you are aggressive towards an additional person, you temporarily feel relief, but then reality kicks in as you feel more stressed out from hurting the other person.

You have to learn ways to manage your

stress and not let it get the better of you and the people around you. Stress drives us to take action but it usually works against us. Here's some of the greatest ways and techniques to manage stress:
1) Leave other people alone - If the other individual is not involved, leave them alone. It is so appealing to release your stress on other people. Don't treat people inappropriately. By treating them the way they don't want to be treated, you build up their stress which they will be joyful to put back on you. If somebody is causing stress, you have to address the person explaining to them how you feel, why you feel that way, and what could be done to solve the problem.
2) Responsiblity - Whenever you take obligation, you live in truth. You don't turn into a victim of others. You start to control and create your feelings. You stop blaming others for what has happened to you and you become proactive controlling thoughts, feelings, and stresses. By

accepting obligation as way of managing stress, you start self-control.

3) Stop worrying - worrying is incredibly dangerous for your health. By worrying you increase the chances of having a heart-attack and you become miserable which damages your relationships. Worrying is about anticipating what's to come and doing nothing about it. If you did do something in anticipation of the future, you'd then be planning and not worrying. You try to think what will happen in the near future, but nothing more then unnecessary thoughts occur. "What if..." "What will happen..." . STOP LIVING IN THE FUTURE and think about what you could fully control now. That is, think about today!

4) Self-control - You are in complete control of your inner thoughts. Its learning to manage your brain that you correctly manage your stress. This is where your self discipline kicks in. Other people don't have

access to your brain unless you give them the authorisation. You have complete control of your inner thoughts and measures . Nonetheless, you're potential to be in control of your inner thoughts and measures is dependent on your desire, discipline, and skill set.

5) Self comprehending - You have to manage your self and control your inner thoughts. You have to be aware if you are treating a person in an applicable way since of the stress. You have to know that you are stressed out, why you are pressured, and ways to manage the stress.

6) Don't stay still - When feeling down, it is uncomplicated to throw in the towel and give up. Winston Churchill stated "If you're going through hell, keep going." Don't stop and give up. I motivate you to stop, calm down, and be smart, but don't lose the perserverance to keep going. If you're going through a bad patch in life, by stopping there you stay in the bad patch.

7) Get away - You might just need to go

away for a bit to refresh your brain. If you could afford a holiday, go for it! For those who can't do that, go for a walk or workout. By being active you release hormones that counteract stress. Additionally, by being away from the stress it clears your brain by taking it away from the problem. Stress is not meant to make us miserable. We are given the potential to produce stress to complete tasks otherwise we would be sitting on our lazy backsides. Learn these ways to manage your stress, and you'll have stress working for you and not you for it.

Chapter 6: Depression: The Basics

Depression and anxiety are two of the most common mental disorders that affect many people. These mental conditions occur as a complicated set of functional or emotional challenges. Both differ in terms of signs and symptoms though in most cases, they tend to occur together. Thus, if you suffer from anxiety, you are likely to develop depression and vice versa, meaning that studying the two conditions is important.

Depression is a common disorder that affects over 350 million people globally. Here in United States, the condition has increased rapidly such that one out of ten people experiences a depressive episode. So, what exactly is depression? Depression in simple terms means a mood disorder that may result in persistent sadness, low-self esteem, or lose of interest. Other terms that best describe the disorder include major depressive disorder, major depression or clinical depression. You need to understand that depression isn't just a normal weakness but a serious health problem. You cannot simply wish it off.

Generally, women are 70 percent more likely to experience depression as compared to men, though both genders experience depression differently. Men tend to experience anger and restlessness and may eventually resort to drugs or alcohol for solitude. Women on the other hand tend to experience guilt or sadness.

Despite depression being blamed for causing suicide, only about 50 percent of people seek treatment, leading to unnecessary suffering that could be eliminated through treatment.

While you may know what depression is, how can you know that you suffer from depression?

Do you Suffer from Depression?

Depression is mainly characterized with low self –esteem, loss of interest in enjoyable activities or low energy and mood. The funny thing is that some depressed people don't really feel sad at all. Instead, they may for instance experience other related symptoms such as being restless, feeling fatigued or being empty. However, experiencing fatigue doesn't always translate to depression.

If you experience persistent conditions such as suicidal thoughts, you could be suffering from major depression. This begs the question; how can you differentiate depression from other related mood disorders? Commons signs and symptoms include:

*Lack of sleep or over sleeping

*Having persistent feelings of hopelessness or helplessness

*Inability to speak, think or move your body freely

*Feeling tired most of the time, without a reason

*Persistent thoughts to commit suicide, thoughts of death or attempted suicide

*Having problems trying to make decisions, concentrate, think, or remember things

*Eating problems such as lack of appetite, food cravings associated with weight loss or weight gain

*Feelings of anger, sadness, frustration, emptiness or irritability over small matters

*Restlessness, agitation, and being anxious. This is characterized by excessive worrying or inability to sit still.

*Loss of interest, feeling guilty and blaming yourself for irrelevant things

The symptoms that you are likely to suffer from will depend on the kind of depression you are suffering from. As such, it is important to know the different types of depression.

Types of Depression

As depression symptoms vary per person, depression types also vary based on symptoms you experience, the duration it occurs and the trigger factors. Let us look at the common types of depression.

Major Depression

The condition is also referred to as major depressive disorder, and causes disabling effects that inhibit proper functioning of your body. Serious symptoms associated with major depression include lack of energy, hopelessness, trouble concentrating, feelings of guilt, and changes in sleep or eating habits, irritability, extreme sadness, and thoughts of death or suicide.

In order to go for diagnosis, your symptoms should persist for about two weeks. In some cases, you may experience one episode or repeated occurrences throughout your entire life.

Mild Chronic Depression

This type of depression is also known as dysthymia, and causes a loss of mood over a long period, for a couple of years, and often longer. These symptoms are not as serious, as in major depression though your body may not function normally. Mild chronic depression can sometimes be characterized with major depression symptoms at one point of life. For diagnosis to confirm that you have this condition, you should experience the symptoms for about 2 years.

Postpartum Depression

This type of depression is also known as postnatal depression or PND and mostly develops within a year after giving birth. However, as opposed to 'baby blues' which lasts for a few days, this condition lasts for up to months or even 2 years in some cases. This condition is characterized by fears about hurting the baby, hopelessness, loneliness, fatigue, extreme sadness and feelings of disconnect from the child. About 10 to 15 percent of all women are reported to experience postnatal depression with the worst part being that in most cases, the condition is not diagnosed and thus goes on without treatment.

SAD (seasonal affective disorder)

You could be among the 4-6 percent of American citizens estimated to suffer from this condition. SAD is characterized by anxiety-like symptoms, daytime fatigue, increased irritability and weight gain. This condition is mostly triggered by winter seasons where there is lesser sunlight, and can be easily treated with light therapy. Symptoms of this condition usually go away during spring or summer.

Psychotic Depression

The term psychosis means a mental condition characterized by hallucinations, such as false sights or sounds, or delusions, best described as false beliefs. This condition is also known as delusional depression. In extreme cases, the condition may become catatonic, where you are totally unable to move, speak, or do other activity.

Bipolar Disorder

The condition is also known as manic-depressive illness, and was formerly known as manic depression. Though it isn't as common as other depression types, it's characterized by extreme lows and highs, known as manias. Its signs and symptoms include excitement, poor judgment, racing thoughts and high energy. These symptoms may alternate between mania and depression a number of times a year.

So, what could be the causes of depression? Let us find out next.

Chapter 7: Discovery Of Thought Field Therapy And Emotional Freedom Technique

Thought Field Therapy (TFT) was developed in 1981 by Roger J Callahan Ph. D, a clinical psychologist.

Roger Callahan found that by tapping the energy points (Meridians) of the body, in a specific sequence, this could balance the body's energy system and eliminate most negative emotions within minutes and promote the body's own healing ability.

Emotional Freedom Technique (EFT) was developed in the 1990's by Gary Craig, as a derivative of TFT. EFT still uses tapping of the energy points (Meridians) as a means to balance the body's energy system and eliminate most negative emotions within minutes.

The main difference between the two systems is;

TFT – uses a specific sequence of tapping for each emotional issue

EFT – uses only one sequence of tapping for all emotional issues

It might be hard to believe but the ideas behind EFT have existed for thousands of years. EFT is based on the subtle energy system of Acupuncture Meridians which was discovered by the Chinese about 5,000 years ago.

More recently, Albert Einstein, told us that everything is composed of energy. Currently, Quantum Theory supports these discoveries.

All forms of positive energy energize us. This energy is transported throughout our body via acupuncture meridians. Sometimes this energy can be disrupted, and we experience its effects: unease, discomfort and pain. With physical tapping at specific points along our energy meridians, EFT "taps" into our energy system to balance it and keep it running smoothly.

Gary Craig stated that "The cause of all negative emotions is a disruption in the body's energy system."

Therefore by tapping specific energy meridians, we can clear the disruptions and bring the body's energy system back into balance.

EFT and the Tapping Points

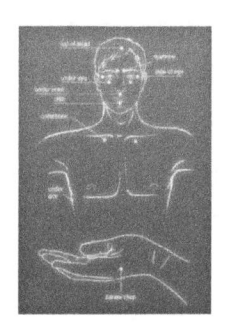

The above diagram shows you the 9 points that we will use to clear all energy disturbances with EFT. The 9 points address all 14 meridians due to the fact that some of the points are located at the intersection of two meridians. Since we are tapping on all meridians when we do EFT, we don't have to worry about which meridians have the disturbance in them. We are tapping on all of the meridians anyway.

See the tapping points diagram. The names of the points starting at the top of the head and going down the body are:

top of head • beginning of eyebrow • side of eye •under eye under nose • chin • collar bone • under arm • karate chop

How to Tap on the Tapping Points

1. Top of the head;

Use all your fingers to "pat" the top of your head so that you don't have to worry about the exact location of the point.

2. All the facial points;

Use two fingers on each point for the same reason.

3. Collar bone point;

The collar bone points are located just below the "knobs" at the end of each collar bone. Use a flat fist just below your neck, where a man would knot his tie, to get one or both of the collar bone points.

4. Under arm point;

This point is located on the side of your body a few inches below your armpit. On a man it is level with the nipple. On a woman it is located in the middle of her bra band. Use all four fingers running up and down on the side of your body to tap on this point.

5. Karate chop point;

The last point on the pinky side of your hand is called the "karate chop" point because it is the place on your hand you would hit if you did a karate chop. You can tap this point any way that you like.

Note:

For the points that are located on both sides of your body, it does not matter which side you use. It's also okay to switch sides while tapping or use both sides simultaneously. It will work any way that you do it.

The tapping on each point should be rapid little "thuds." You should tap hard enough to feel some percussion during each tap but not hard enough that you will begin to feel tender after a lot of tapping. You only need to tap each point around 4 to 6 times, though more is not a problem. You won't need to count taps because you will be saying a phrase at each point (see below). Just tap rapidly while saying the phrase, and that will be enough taps.

Chapter 8: What Is Stress?

Stress is a word that is often heard and talked about but truly, not fully understood. Some people consider stress as an event that happens in their lives, like losing a job or experiencing an accident or injury. Some people on the other hand would say that stress is the behavior of the body towards certain events such as nail biting or anxiety.

In actuality, stress involves both the event and response of the body and mind to the so-called stressor (source of stress). When a person undergoes a situation, it is automatically evaluated by the mind mentally. The mind decides if the situation is a threat then generates logic on how to deal with the situation at hand and if the person has the skill to solve the problem. If it is decided that the skills acquired by the person is not enough to handle the problem, then the situation is labeled "stressful". If the situation is something the person can handle, then it is considered otherwise.

There are many sources of stress. Contrary to common belief, it is not always sourced from a negative situation. It could also be caused by positive situations like a job promotion or a new baby. The body experiences stress even in these positive changes, because it has to adapt to new challenges. For some people, being flooded with added work and activities could cause enormous stress. Another good example of a positive situation that can cause stress is pregnancy or giving birth. For a mother especially that is experiencing pregnancy for the first time, the body experiences enormous change. These changes may cause imbalances on the body, therefore releasing stress hormones. When the baby is born, both the father and mother will experience changes in their lifestyle, if not properly conditioned for these changes, the situation also triggers stress.

Negative situations on the other hand such as loss of a loved one or being fired from a job causes stress resulting from emotional instability. Negative situations are considered more stressful other people would say but actually it is not. The level of stress felt by a person would not depend on the situation or the stressor but it would also depend on the ability of the body and mind to handle these stressors.

Since stress is acquired when the body and mind are weak and cannot handle threats, keeping it stronger and more resilient to stressors definitely prevents people from being stressed out. If stress cannot be prevented, techniques that can help people cope with stress can be done.

This book will explain how these techniques should be helpful in coping with stress and how it can make people handle stressful situations with grace and calm.

Chapter 9: Understanding Depression

Depression is a psychological disorder that exhibits low mood, despair, sadness, self-reproach, low self-esteem, and loneliness. This condition can be manifested by people who disengage from any social contact, possess psychomotor retardation, and have a diminishing appetite. While depression has gained a deeper understanding from the scholars' point of view, many people still treat this condition as a normal phase in every individual's life without considering its possible long-term implications. A good understanding of this condition can help a person cope with the adverse effects.

According to studies, depression can be caused by an individual's natural environment, genes, personal experiences, drug abuse, alcohol problems, bad lifestyle, and/or specific life events. Take note that a great deal of psychological factors effect a person's mood and emotions; thus, personal life experiences such as one's menopausal period, financial problems, heartbreaks, and bereavement can contribute to this condition. Some studies also relate depression to existing non-psychiatric disorders such as Addison's disease, sleep apnea, and multiple sclerosis. Some cases cite depression as one of the early symptoms of an existing medical condition where a person may feel restless, sad, irritable, low, lonely, hopeless, empty, and worthless. Those who are prone to suicidal tendencies are often said to be suffering from depression as well.

The impact of depression may vary from one person to another. For example, several reports assert that depression among women is twice as high as that of men. This is partly because of some hormonal factors (e.g. Pre-Menstrual Syndrome) that are prevalent in women. In addition, depression may be classified according to the factors that constitute the entire condition. The different types of depression include Major Depression, Dysthymia, and Seasonal Affective Disorder. Depending on the intensity of the case, depression may be treated in a wide variety of ways including seeking professional help through therapy sessions. This treatment allows the person suffering from depression to determine the cause of the condition using psychological and physiological parameters, which will eventually lead to developing skills in coping with the condition.

Change in lifestyle habits may also bring positive effects to the depressed patient. Another way to treat depression is by taking vitamins and other food supplements to help alleviate any possible chemical imbalance. Psychotherapy, electric shock treatments, and acupuncture, on the other hand, can also be considered as an alternative to medication. A person can also resort to antidepressants and other medications in combating the condition. Selective Serotonin Reuptake Inhibitors (SSRIs) are one of the latest antidepressants offered in the medical field. It makes use of serotonin as the main ingredient in fighting the symptoms and effects of depression.

Chapter 10: All You Need To Know About Social Anxiety And Social Phobia

The characteristics are there, subtle but visible, if you look closely.

There are the introverted people, shying away from unknown company. They worry about what people would think about them, they worry about the way they dress sometimes, they are anxious about approaching people they don't know. They blush when speaking to people of the opposite sex, they stutter when speaking in public, they mutter and whisper. They are the timid ones, the introverts, the withdrawn people.

And then there are some people whose shyness seem just too much to others; you can never be sure whether they are really like that, or just making it up.

These people are seen to be excessively and unreasonably afraid of social situations. They are always under the intense fear that they would be negatively judged and criticized by others. They lack social skills and are afraid they will make mistakes and be laughed at almost every waking moment of their life. This is 'Social Anxiety'.

And this is fact, not an exaggeration. There are millions of people in this world who are living their lives with social anxiety.

Social Anxiety is sometimes known as Social Phobia, or Social Anxiety Disorder, and is mainly characterized by an unhealthy and irrational fear of judgment, criticism and embarrassment. People suffering from Social phobia are afraid to face any kind of social situations and they would avoid confrontations and interactions at the cost of their own welfare.

Social Anxiety is more common in women than men, and more in children and youngsters compared to adults. It generally starts as early as childhood, or adolescent and persists until the person is aware of the problem and seeks help. However, even after full understanding of their situation or setback, very few people are willing to look for treatment or help due to fear of being ridiculed and humiliated, which makes recovery more difficult.

Social Phobia is present all over the world, and is the most common mental illness in the United States, affecting more than 40 million adults in the country.

Causes of Social Anxiety

The causes of Social Anxiety in people may be many, diverse and varying from person to person. These causes may be genetic or environmental and can generally be categorized into five.

<u>Inheritance:</u> Children raised by parent(s) who suffer from Social Anxiety themselves, or are of a nervous and introvert manner, can result in a high chance of developing Social Phobia/Anxiety themselves. This condition

tends to run in families, both by heredity as well as learned behavior.

Brain Structure and Chemistry: Amygdala is a structure in the brain that causes fear response in a person. A human being who has a vigorous Amygdala is more prone to feeling anxious and nervous in public. Besides, serotonin is a chemical whose imbalance in the human brain is known to cause social anxiety disorder.

Family Conflict: Children growing up in families with longstanding conflict and internal problems often grow up to be nervous, anxious and tensed. Since their families failed to provide a safe environment for them while growing up, they usually view the whole world as a dangerous place where everyone will always judge, humiliate and criticize them.

Negative Experience: People who have suffered from any kind of negative experience in their life such as bullying, sexual and physical abuse, rape and molestation as a child, regular fear and living in terror, even constant teasing from siblings and parents, rejection or humiliation can sometimes develop social anxiety and fear of facing anyone or opening up to anyone.

Geographical Location: Surprisingly, some studies show that people living in warmer weather and higher population density, such as the Mediterranean countries are less in risk of social anxiety disorder than people living in colder and less populated regions, like the Scandinavian countries of Europe.

These five categories sum up the reasons why some people may develop social anxiety disorder in their childhood or adolescent years. Of course, there may be some other reasons since every human being in this world is unique, and complex. Also, just because these reasons have been identified as the grounds behind social anxiety, it is not that every person who goes through these situations will develop social phobia.

Who is at Risk?

As with any other disorders, there are specific groups of people who are more at risk than others. For Social anxiety disorder, I have categorized them into five groups.

<u>By Sex:</u> **Females are more at risk of developing social phobia than males.**

<u>By Age:</u> **Children, teenagers and adolescents are more prone to develop social anxiety disorder than a person who is well into their 30s or 40s.**

<u>By Temperament:</u> **People who were naturally shy, timid or withdrawn during their childhood or teenage years are more likely to become socially anxious when meeting new people or facing new environments.**

By Health Condition: Growing up with a health condition, especially if the condition was visible and kept them separated from their peers, such as a limp, facial disfigurement, scars, stuttering, etc can trigger social phobia in people.

Children with such physical conditions are often bullied on and teased by their peers during their early years, causing them to withdraw into themselves and fear social situations.

By Family Background: **Children growing up with parents, siblings or extended family members who has social anxiety disorder are also in the risk of developing this phobia themselves.**

By Parenting Technique: **Some experts believe that children who have over-protective parents, i.e. parents who are always anxious and worried about their children's wellbeing and progress, are at a risk of developing social anxiety disorder.**

As with the causes behind Social Anxiety, the points mentioned above do not mean that any individual or children in these situations will definitely develop this disorder, but they are definitely at a higher risk than others.

Chapter 11: How Can Tapping Benefit You?

By correctly implementing EFT and tapping techniques in your daily life and practicing it on a regular basis, you can reap a lot of benefits. Tapping improves general overall health and can also be used to overcome physical problems.

It helps in mitigating and alleviating pain.

It helps you to calm down and relax and which can help you get good sleep (this works in treating sleeping related ailments like insomnia). This can also help you handle unpleasant situations and maintain an emotionally balanced life.

It can positively influence your emotions and encourage you to adopt healthy diet plans. This works by helping to reduce or get rid of cravings.

EFT helps to block negative feelings and help you find happiness. This helps you accept and love yourself just the way you are which is a sure fire way to boost self-esteem.

It is also found to be effective for different psychological conditions as listed below:

a) Helps to overcome emotional issues like stress and anxiety. By reducing stress, you would be able to work well and improve the productivity at workplace. EFT also helps to deal with depression.

b) It has also been found to be an effective treatment for different types of phobias, whether it's social anxiety or fears like arachnophobia.

c) It is also effective in overcoming addictions, whether it's food or alcohol. People suffering from Obsessive-compulsive disorder can use EFT as a good therapy.

d) EFT also helps to treat different physical issues like irritable bowel syndrome, fertility issues, and can help combat allergies and rashes.

e) EFT can also be used in children to help remove fears or phobias. It could also help students suffering from school phobia and help them to deal with learning and behavioral difficulties. Tapping can also act as an effective step to beat the bully.

Why tapping is efficient compared to other treatments or therapies?

Tapping is a reliable and pain-free method of treatment, unlike treatments like acupuncture. You don't need to undergo any kind of surgical procedures or use any medication. Tapping is also an affordable method of treatment. There are plenty of videos available online which will allow you to learn and practice this technique from the comfort of your home. There is a large following of this method of treatment, which implies that this method is quite effective as well.

EFT helps to nurture love for yourself; in this method, you get to know more about your own personal strong points and flaws. It will help you accept your flaws and this makes it easy to work on the problems and encourage you to overcome them instead of criticizing and blaming yourself. Our mind and body function best witha positive mind-set which can be achieved through positive statements or affirmations, which forms the basis of this psychological treatment method. Using these affirmations will help you slowly, but surely, affect your brain in a positive way. This will allow you to grow and get the positive results you desire.

Now that you've learned about all the wonderful benefits of EFT let's look at how it works in the next chapter.

Chapter 12: How Can Aromatherapy Help To Reduce Anxiety?

Aromatherapy can be a useful tool in combating anxiety. It is a natural remedy to help ease symptoms. Essential oils and calming herbs can be used to alleviate major anxiety symptoms. The benefits include physical, emotional and spiritual well-being. Including scents from essential oils in a regular routine, over time, can alleviate anxiety all together.

In addition to aromatherapy, anxiety sufferers can also introduce a caffeine free/sugar free lifestyle, a healthy diet, and regular exercise to counteract anxiety. All of these things, combined with aromatherapy will increase the likelihood of living an anxiety free life and will enhance the feelings of tranquility.

Aromatherapy for anxiety can help one to embrace their thoughts with comfort and softness and at the same time, embrace feelings. This is a science of translating smell of the aroma to a positive thought of what the oil reminds us of. Your sense of smell has the capability of traveling into the part of the limbic brain that is the base of our emotions and memories.

Using aromatherapy for anxiety in the bath, just like with stress, is the easiest and most pleasant way to benefit from it. A simple technique of taking an aromatic bath can be quite relaxing. Several studies show that Lavender aromatherapy helps relieve anxiety. These studies show the possibility that aromatherapy for anxiety may affect mood, cognitive performance and relaxation. However, more studies need to be done to confirm this information.

Chapter 13: What Is Anxiety?

According to the Anxiety and Depression Association of America, anxiety affects 18% of adults in America alone. An individual with anxiety is three to five times more likely to visit a doctor and six times more likely to be hospitalized in a psych ward than the average person. About 1/3 of the U.S.'s health fund goes towards helping those with anxiety disorders.

Although anxiety can be caused by a variety of factors, stress is a major factor that fuels anxiety. The Mayo Clinic supports this theory, citing examples of stress buildup or stress due to an illness. Stress buildup happens during an accumulation of smaller stressors in your life like financial problems, relational conflicts, or traffic. Stress due to having an illness or having a family member with an illness can trigger worry about the future and can cause anxiety.

Anxiety is an excessive feeling of worry, nervousness, apprehension, and dread. It can vary in intensity. Mild anxiety usually causes a feeling of uneasiness and apprehension. Severe anxiety can hamper one's ability to function, sleep, or work. Some anxiety is normal, however, if anxiety lingers and starts to affect your productivity at work or in your daily tasks, you might have a more serious case of anxiety that would necessitate seeing a health professional.

Chapter 14: The F-E-A-R-L-E-S-S Mantra

Conquering your fears makes you feel empowered, courageous, and proud and free. So be your own 'fear-therapist'. Reprogram your brain by swearing to the F-E-A-R-L-E-S-S mantra and feel your fears fading away.

F – Face your Fears

Begin by acknowledging and owning up to your fears.

Name your fears be it tangible ones or those lurking in the back of your mind.

Write down your fears and officially admit that you have a problem you want to overcome. **Keeping a journal** is even a better way to track your progress as you work toward conquering your fear. Also, use it for your reference the next time fear comes your way.

E – Erase Negative Imprints

In order to do so, first define the contours of your fears. Give a shape to your fear by marking its beginning and an end; this equips you to contain and control your fears better.

Many times, your fears stem from your own negative experiences or from witnessing the hardships of those around you. Figure out exactly what power your fear has over your mind and behavior.

Think about the history of your fear.

Did it begin with a negative experience? Is it related to factors that affected your childhood environment? - Your fear of divorce may very well be rooted in your own parents' divorce.

For how long have you been affected by this fear?

What triggers your fear till date? Does the idea of marriage or even dating trigger the fear of divorce in you?

How does your fear affect you? Are you commitment phobic? Do you detest the idea of having kids with your partner? Do you feel restless while attending social gatherings such as marriages and escape at the first presented opportunity?

Write down the answers to these questions and the read the answers out loud. These answers will help you remind yourself that your past is past and non-existent anymore, therefore , its mental imprints has to be removed permanently in order to free your mind.

A – Anticipate and Allow Change

Now that you completely understand your fear, think about what and how much exactly you want to change.

Even if the change may seem to uproot you from your comfort zone and hence frightening at first, you must allow necessary changes to come your way. Set small concrete goals that will help you transport yourself into a new greater manifestation of yourself.

For example,

If your fear is enclosed spaces, you could start by taking a lift to travel just one floor of a building like your apartment or your friend's apartment.

If you are commitment phobic, your first concrete goal may be to date someone for longer than a month.

You must consciously and gradually dethrone "security" and replace it with the active virtue of "courage."

R – Reframe your fears

Nothing gets our hearts racing like a little harmless terror—so why not harness what frightens you to make your life richer?

What about the roller coaster ride that you took last time? Sure you were scared but can you contest the excitement that you experienced? Don't you want to take that roller coaster ride again just for that sheer feeling of thrill?

Treat your fears as opportunities for experiencing adventures and explorations.

When you feel fear of something unfamiliar, take it as a sign that you need to get to know a person or situation better. If you are afraid of heights, think about the possibilities that will be open to you once you overcome the fear; you can travel around the world and enjoy sports like bungee jumping

Try confronting your fear with this new perspective in mind. View fear in a positive

light, view it as a source of energy. Does it feel any different? Can you embrace its role in your life now?

L – Let fear have a place in your life

Fear builds character and teaches us how to act with courage. We would live with reckless abandon if we knew no notion of fear, performing all sorts of downright dangerous activities. The key is to distinguish between actions, which induce a healthy acknowledgment of apprehension versus illogical triggers of fear, which stifle our potential and limit our well-being.

E – Encounter your fears

If mystery scares you, try gradual desensitization by exposing yourself to it in small doses until you gain a better understanding and your fear begins to dissipate. For instance, if you are afraid of spiders, start by looking at a badly drawn cartoon of a spider done in silly colors. When you succeed in controlling your reactions, move up to photos of spiders. Finally, try cleaning up dead spiders.

Consider direct confrontation particularly you are afraid of a particular person or situation. Imagine the worst-case scenario. What's the worst that could happen if you made an appointment with your dentist to fix that tooth of yours? If you know you'll come out on the other side alive, well and proud of your achievement, go for it.

S – Stick to the Momentum

It takes a certain amount of momentum to deal with fear. It's essential that you take time out for yourself to relax, calm down but stick to the momentum. Remember the golden saying – "Slow and Steady wins the race." Stay determined to persevere even when you face setbacks.

Resist the temptation to hope things turn out for the best and leave it up to fate. Always keep in mind that you have control of your future. You have the power to determine the path you will take.

Recognize when other people try to hold you back and don't let them succeed in their intentions. Rather surround yourself with people and thoughts (from books, television shows, movies) that will help you overcome your fears and reach your potential.

S – Secure in Yourself

In order to shun fear forever, you have to work on your self-esteem. Fear arises from not believing enough in your own abilities and talents. When you constantly live in the mindset of "I can't do it" or, "I'm not good enough," you narrow your window of success to a very slim opening and inadvertently put yourself down.

Confronting a fear is hard, and it doesn't always lead to a triumphant conclusion. So be prepared to deal with failure. Work on your self-esteem; don't let the fear of failure prevent you from believing enough in your own abilities and talents. Thrive in the positive mindset of: "I can do it; I shall prove that I am good enough at this". Face your fears as many times as required before you can declare it conquered, and shun fear forever.

However, do not wait to shun your fear for good so that you can give yourself a pat on the back. Rather celebrate each milestone. Share your stories with people at a party or an even wider audience through blogs. Once you get the taste of appreciation for your smaller victories, you'll be ready to face your next conquest.

Chapter 15: Principles Of Meditation

Despite the differences in the types of meditation, each of them is founded on specific qualities/principles, which must be present if the needed level of meditation is to be attained, which will in turn bring the varied benefits. Some of these qualities/features or principles include:

Relaxed Breathing

In any meditation technique, your pace of breathing determines how easy it would be to enter into the space between your thoughts and attain calmness and peace that meditation is all about. Breathing for meditation should be even paced and deep entailing the use of diaphragm muscles to expand or relax your lungs. You have to ensure you get enough oxygen while ensuring that you reduce the movement of upper chest muscles, neck and shoulders to enhance efficiency in your breathing.

Being Fully Focused

Your ability to focus all your attention greatly influences your success rate in any meditation exercise; it is one of the core elements of meditation. This will help your mind to get into a state of calmness where distractions, stresses and worries don't exist. It could entail focusing on a flame of a candle, focusing on repeating a mantra or focusing on your breath in a bid to attain calmness of mind that you get when you are at a state of pure consciousness where you interact with your innermost self.

A Quite Setting

It can be almost impossible to meditate in an area with too many distractions around you especially if you are starting out. Regardless of the type of meditation technique you want to opt for, it is paramount that you find a quiet spot to focus your attention. With continuous practice, it will be much easier to meditate even when you are in highly distractive environments.

A Comfortable Position

You certainly cannot meditate unless you are in a comfortable sitting, upright, lying, walking or other position. Being comfortable is key to getting rid of the distractions around you to make it through the zone of pure consciousness where you experience calmness, tranquility and peace irrespective of the surroundings.

Although many people try to meditate (through fixing their thoughts in one area for a long time), many actually never succeed in making it a repetitive activity. It is the frequency and consistency that will produce the biggest impact for good feelings in the long term to help fight anxiety, enhance concentration and improve a feeling of self happiness. Having the right mindset to make meditation a sustainable practice can make a big difference in succeeding in your efforts to meditate in order to fight stress, anxiety and depression by getting to a state of pure consciousness where distractive or unhappy thoughts have no place. As a beginner, you need to put into consideration a number of points if you are to learn any meditation technique and achieve the value you hope to achieve through your efforts. Getting past the initial challenges is the key to making meditation part of your everyday life.

Chapter 16: Therapy For Panic Attacks

And Anxiety

Anxiety can have very unpleasant consequences if left untreated. Aside from panic attacks, it can also lead to a variety of health conditions. If you suffer from anxiety and panic attacks and yet you still refuse to seek treatment immediately, your symptoms can get worse and make even the simplest tasks difficult to accomplish.

Recurring panic attacks, for instance, may cause you to confine yourself to your home and never go out. Your fear of having another panic attack can cost you your job, studies, and personal relationships. You can also develop depression and other psychological disorders.

You may turn to alcohol or illegal drugs and eventually become addicted to the substance. If this happens, you will have more problems and you will only find it harder to bounce back. You should realize that addiction can also affect your family, especially in terms of finances and other responsibilities.

Fortunately, you can get treatment for your panic attacks and anxiety. Psychotherapy, for instance, is an ideal option. Sessions usually last for several months. According to the National Health Service, working with a trained therapist can help you view your problems and worries in a more positive perspective.

Psychotherapy sessions can also include music, art, and drama to make you more at ease in expressing your thoughts and emotions. Your therapist can use a variety of techniques based on behavior change, communication, relationship building, and dialogue.

Cognitive Behavioral Therapy

Cognitive behavioral therapy is a very popular treatment for anxiety disorders. In fact, it is the most favored form of treatment for panic attack, panic disorder, and agoraphobia. It focuses on the behavior and thinking patterns of the patient so he may be able to deal with his fears in a realistic manner.

Cognitive behavioral therapy involves working with a psychologist to help the patient identify and deal with the factors that may have caused his anxiety. It also involves techniques that can significantly reduce or stop certain behaviors that cause him to be more anxious.

In a cognitive behavioral therapy session, your therapist will ask you to relax, breathe deeply, and find out how your thoughts can cause you to experience symptoms of panic attacks or anxiety. You should be able to identify the thought patterns that trigger your panic attacks. Once you are able to do this, you will be asked to try to change your thought patterns so you can avoid experiencing these symptoms again.

The psychologists who administer cognitive behavioral therapy usually combine behavioral techniques with cognitive awareness to help patients tolerate and confront stressful situations in a safe and controlled environment. They can also combine it with medications.

Interpersonal Therapy

You may also undergo interpersonal therapy, which involves helping patients deal with personal relationships that are difficult and causing them to be depressed. If you undergo interpersonal therapy, you may also be allowed to combine it with medications for a speedier recovery.

Exposure Therapy

If you frequently have panic attacks, you can undergo exposure therapy and be exposed to various physical sensations of panic. This treatment is typically done in a safe and controlled environment, so you can rest assured that you will be able to cope quickly. Therapy sessions may involve shaking your head, hyperventilating, or holding your breath.

You need to do these exercises because they mimic the actual symptoms of a panic attack. Each time you are exposed to such sensations, you get used to them. This allows you to reduce your fear of experiencing the symptoms of a panic attack and be able to control yourself better.

Chapter 17: Realize, Accept And Manage

Most of the girls of her age would go out with their friends, shop in the mall, travel around the world, but not her. She would rather stay in her room, read her books and study for her class. Upon waking up, she would take a bath, eat her breakfast, and go to school. In school, she would attentively listen to her professor, take a break for lunch, and go to the library after class where she spends a couple of hours of her time to read books. When she comes home, she would go up to her room, take a nap for 20 minutes, eat dinner, and study again. She does this every day, except for weekends, of course, when she doesn't go to school.

One time, when she wasn't able to follow her routine, she suddenly felt anxious. From then on, she kept on looking at her wristwatch, checking the time every now and then, looking at her calendar every so often to check her schedule. She would open her journal and cross and uncross her activities, not knowing what to do first or what to do last. She would sometimes shout at her little brother for being noisy that she couldn't concentrate on her tasks. She would reject the calls of her friends irritably and would ignore the calls of her mom. She would usually miss the fun of family outings and class parties.

Most people would have this kind of safety zone, a routine where they feel comfortable and complacent enough to get them through the day. Just like the girl in the story, people have a routine that they don't want to break, a routine that they faithfully follow. Most people do what the girl does. They fill their calendars with their schedules, mark the dates of their deadlines and time all their activities, from the time of waking up to the time before they sleep. Routines could be nice because they give you the sense of familiarity, but the problem with routines is that once they get broken, all the bad things in the world seem to break loose. People become anxious, restless, and annoyed.

It is good to have a list of all the activities or tasks that you need to accomplish. It's a way of time management and it is a way of checking how far you've gone from your starting point. But too much reliance on your schedule can make you lonely. You may not feel right away, but the people around you would surely see and feel it. Don't be afraid to try out other things and take a slice of freedom. Time is too short to be spent on things that you can't cherish in the end. Yes, it's true that the results of your hard work are something to be proud of. But when you look back at the times that you have spent on them, you might not feel any emotion at all.

A preacher once said that when you recall the times when you have been busy doing all sorts of things, you won't remember anything about it. Why? This is because you were doing everything like a robot.

There was nothing worth remembering. All you can remember would be the days you have spent on finishing your tasks, the times you have spent beating the deadlines, and the moments you have spent trying to fit everything into your calendar. You may think that those times were productive, but when you look back on them, you'll feel empty. You'll only remember the hardships but no happiness. All for the sake of staying in your comfort zone.

Anxiety can sometimes get the best of you, ruin the days that should have been your greatest moments, and deprive you of your happiness. There are a lot of events, factors and triggers that can cause anxiety and it is best if you equip yourself with the different ways on how to fight it off.

1. Get to know yourself.

When trying to fight off a stressor, the first step is always getting to know yourself. Know what causes you stress, what you hate most, and what you like doing most. Know what works for you and what doesn't. If writing a journal helps you relieve you off your stress, then write it. If singing is what works for you best, then sing at the top of your lungs. In reality, there's nothing wrong or right when choosing what works for you and what doesn't. It's just a matter of doing things in moderation and choosing the "right" one – that is, the one that is most appropriate for the situation. If you have a deadline to beat and you are getting stressed about it, singing a song or two is fine. But don't sing all night long if the deadline is tomorrow! And you will know what is best for you if you know yourself well.

2. Accept that you have limitations.

Fears and worries usually spring out from the inability of a person to accept that one cannot do everything. Acceptance of one's limitations is the cornerstone in formulating your solutions. If you deny that there is a problem, this problem will just keep on haunting you. Running away or ignoring the problem doesn't solve it. Recognize that though you can't do everything, you can definitely do SOMETHING. Learn to be flexible in the face of your limitations.

3. Manage it.

The last step in overcoming your anxiety is solving it. Face it and fight it head on. You can't proceed to the next stages or next phases of your life if you keep on avoiding it. Moving forward is different from beating around the bush. Avoiding or running away from your problem doesn't keep you away from it, rather it just keeps you moving in circles.

If you are anxious about a future event, prepare for it. If you are anxious about not being able to keep your job, do your best in everything that you have to do. If your boss sees that you are working hard, he will definitely think twice about firing you. If you are anxious about the results of your exams, study harder. There are different ways on how to counteract your anxiety. All you have to do is to recognize it and target the source. Just like how you cure a disease, don't treat the symptom, rather, treat the main source. If the disease is caused by the bacteria, kill the microorganisms, not just the pain.

Chapter 18: Group Therapy

Some anxiety sufferers respond very well to being surrounded by individuals going through the same thing they are. Group therapy, in and of itself, can often bring a surprising degree of comfort. It puts in front of you, living, breathing human beings that know exactly what you're going through. You wouldn't believe just how much of a relief it can be to finally be with other men and women who deal with anxiety. <u>You are not alone!</u>

Another benefit to group therapy is the sharing of successful techniques that the members have tried. You can learn things, or share things with the group that they may not have tried yet, or even thought of. This can also alleviate, or greatly reduce, some of the overwhelming feelings of how to move forward with your day-to-day activities.

Interpersonal Therapy

This form of psychotherapy is primarily used with depression but has proven effective with some anxieties. It deals with your relationships with others. Basically, anxiety and its associated conditions can affect relationships and relationships affect mood. How you interact with others while going through anxiety can directly affect how willingly others will deal with you, much less try to help you.

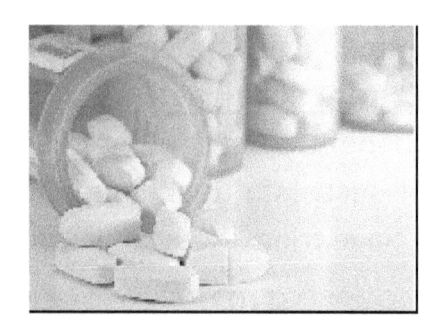

Chapter 19: Turning Relaxation Techniques Into Habits

At this very moment, you are worried about the level of stress that you mind and body are experiencing and you are doing something about it, which is a good thing. However, after reading this book you might find yourself slowly falling into the same trap full of stress and worries. That is why it is important for you to make a lifestyle change and put all of the techniques that you have learned into your daily routine.

Try to recall the last time that you were stressed out. How did you handle it? Did you smoke, drink alcohol, took drugs, watch too much television, or ate too much unhealthy food? Did you lie in bed all day, got mad and lashed out at someone else, or became cold towards your loved ones? All these and more are negative ways of coping with stress and you need to find healthier alternatives to them. To deal with stress, you have two options: to change the situation or to change your attitude towards the situation.

Avoiding Stress

There are times when you can actually avoid unnecessary stress. Learn and practice the art of saying "no". Place a limit on how much you can handle in your work and personal life, and say no to responsibilities which go beyond that limit. You can also stay away from people who cause a lot of stress in your life. Let go of a toxic relationship, distance yourself from negative co-workers, and stay away from hectic environments, such as doing online shopping instead of visiting the mall.

Create a to-do list carefully. Deal with the heavier assignments at the start of the day so that you will feel more relaxed on the latter part of your schedule. Break down big projects into smaller, more manageable tasks. Rank your to-do's based on importance and not urgency.

Resist the urge to have a cup of coffee after 10 AM. While caffeine and sugar might give you that instant boost of energy to deal with a jam-packed schedule, it is one of the main culprits against your much needed rest at the end of the day. Try alternatives, such as green tea in lieu of coffee; it is a healthier choice and it can help you relax. But if you can't help it, then reward yourself with a cup of java just at the break of dawn.

Changing your Attitude

There are times when the situation cannot be avoided, so what you can do instead is to change your attitude towards it. Avoid keeping your feelings pent up inside of you; however, do not unleash it upon a helpless victim. Vent it all out on your stress journal, or share it respectfully with a good friend. After that, let it go and focus on something more productive.

Learn how to stick up for yourself as well. Practice negotiating and being more assertive so that you can take charge of your life instead of letting others make demands from you. But you must also practice being more flexible and be willing to compromise if the situation requires it. Take things positively and do the job well without sacrificing your sanity.

Reassess the standards you have set for others and yourself. Perfectionism is one of the main causes of stress, so it is best to adapt to situations which come out "alright" instead of "perfect." There will always be times when things do not go according to plan, and that is not entirely a bad thing. During these moments, take a step back and ask yourself if this problem will matter next month or next year.

Remind yourself that you cannot always control everything, such as how other people think and behave. Instead of letting the stress of others affect you, take these as an opportunity for you to grow. Choose to forgive, as it is a much more stress-free option than to exact revenge, which can snowball into an even bigger problem in the future.

Make Time for Rest and Relaxation
Everybody deserves some time off after studying and working hard every day. It does not have to be an expensive trip to an exotic beach or a splurge at a luxurious spa, although there's nothing wrong with these if you can afford it. Insert little habits in your daily schedule to allow your body some time to recharge.

Always find the time to reconnect with your loved ones regardless of how busy you week is. Watch a comedy with your spouse, enjoy a bike ride with your best friend, play a board game with your kids, or cuddle up with your dog.

Develop the habit of becoming a morning person. You can accomplish a lot more when you jumpstart your day at 5 in the morning. Go out for an early morning jog and let your happy hormones charge you up for the day. And before you get ready for bed, enjoy a relaxing, warm bath and enjoy a warm cup of herbal tea. It doesn't have to be a routine for you can always find alternatives that are just as relaxing. And, most importantly, never cut back on your sleep.

Chapter 20: Fears And Depression Associated With Narcissistic Abuse

Narcissism lies on a continuum from healthy to pathological. Healthy narcissism is part of normal human functioning. It represents required self - love and confidence based on real achievements and the ability to overcome setbacks.

But, narcissism becomes a problem when one becomes excessively preoccupied with the self and seeks complete admiration and attention, with complete disregard for others' feelings.

Lack of satisfaction of this need leads to substance abuse and major depressive disorders. In adolescents, this causes 'Substance Dependency Disorder' (SDD) - they display overt narcissistic and prosocial behaviors, which show a connection between self - centeredness and addiction.

These substances include sedatives like alcohol, psychedelics and hallucinogens like marijuana and LSD, stimulants like cocaine, narcotics like opium, heroin, and morphine, and anti-anxiety drugs like Xanax.

Narcissists unconsciously deny an unstated and intolerably poor self - image through inflation. They turn themselves into glittering figures of immense grandeur, surrounded by psychologically impenetrable walls. The goal of this self - deception is to be impervious to greatly feared external criticism, and to their own rolling sea of doubts.

The narcissists fail to achieve intimacy with anyone as they view other people like items in a vending machine, and uses them to serve their own needs, never being able to acknowledge that others might have their own feelings too.

Healthy, non - egotistical self - love arises from an unconditional acceptance of the self, without having to declare superiority over others.

Deep down, the narcissists know, albeit unconsciously, that they are not really what they project. In fact, one of their central defenses is to endlessly project onto others the very flaws and fears that they are unable or unwilling, to allow into awareness.

They are critical of others' shortcomings, but completely blind to their own - their self - love must be seen as an illusion, a spectacular triumph of self - deception. They can only love their false, idealized self - a mirage that cannot possibly return the fantasy - laden love.

Their flawed self, hidden beneath their outward bravado, remains locked up and placed in permanent exile. And, to continuously safeguard themselves from a reality that so frequently contradicts their grandiose assumptions and pretensions, they are forced to employ a massive defense stratagem, with extraordinary rigidity.

Although very few of us are actually diagnosed with NPD, almost all of us are guilty of sharing certain narcissistic tendencies. For true narcissists, the defenses are absolutely necessary to compensate their ego deficits and reduce feelings of shame.

Without them, they might result in a state of suicidal depression; for, narcissists do not really like themselves - the more they boast and demean others, they are more likely to cover up for their deeper, largely hidden feelings of inferiority and lack of love.

Blinded by their idealized self - image, they try to project themselves as gifted, exceptional and unique - that in turn makes them egotistical and arrogant. They don't mean to do harm but the harm [that they cause] does not interest them.

Or they do not see it or they justify it because they are absorbed in the endless struggle to think well of themselves." This shows a distinction between narcissists who are malevolent, and those who simply lack concern of how their behavior might adversely affect others. It is yet another way of gaining attention to their supreme self - absorption, which makes it impossible for them to identify with others' feelings.

The 'narcissistic dilemma' is seen when, being criticized, the narcissists show themselves pitifully incapable of retaining any emotional poise or receptivity. But, these disturbed individuals also display an abnormally developed capacity to criticize others.

Their dilemma is that the rigidity of their defenses, their inability ever to let their guard down, even among their closest people, guarantees that they will never get what they most need, which unfortunately, they are themselves oblivious to.

People are never born narcissist, it is powerful environmental influences that make them so. Being neglected and ignored, or constantly disparaged or berated by parents in childhood, they form unrealistically high standards of behavior.

Unable to meet up to their parents' unreasonable, perfectionist expectations, they create an imaginary "ideal self" that could receive the parental acceptance, even adulation, which they yearn for.

The main elements of narcissism are narcissistic supply, narcissistic rage and narcissistic injury, and narcissistic abuse. Narcissism can be of various types, and its causes are not yet well - known. Inherited genetic defects are thought to be responsible in some cases, along with environmental factors -

1. Childhood abuse or neglect
2. Excessive parental pampering
3. Unrealistic expectation from parents
4. Sexual promiscuity
5. Cultural influences

Today, Narcissism has gripped the entire world, as indicated by the rapid change in society that occurred during the industrial and post - industrial times.

The past few decades have witnessed a societal shift from a commitment to the collective to a focus on the individual or self. Here comes in the 'self - esteem movement' which became the key to success in life.

The parents tried to "confer" self - esteem upon their children rather than allowing them to achieve it through hard work. The rise of individualism and the decline in social norms that accompanied the modernization of society, led to a shift from the concept of what is best for the others and family to what is best for "me".

Chapter 21: Why And How To Focus On Others

Often, people with social anxiety don't realize at all that they're focusing most of their attention on themselves. It may seem like you're always thinking of the other person. After all, you're worrying about their reactions to what you say and what they will think of you. But, if you look at these thoughts clearly, you'll realize that your focus isn't on their wants or needs. It's on fear that you won't get what you want and need, namely acceptance and respect. If you want to get over your social anxiety, it's a good idea to make a switch and start thinking about the other person more than you think about yourself.

Why Focus on Others?

You might feel completely justified in focusing on yourself when you're in social situations. After all, it's your problem to deal with, right? Well, yes, it is your problem to take care of, but don't lose sight of the fact that your problem isn't the only one in the room. Everyone has their own challenges in life. When you recognize that others are struggling with their own problems, you feel less alone in the world. When you care about others' problems, you are more likely to be forgiving of the small slights that once made you feel panicked.

When you focus on others, you go beyond your anxious thinking and into a more social consciousness. If you really want to interact with others, you have to meet them halfway. You need to let the experience happen without prejudging it so you can see what this unique individual has to contribute to the conversation.

Focusing on others gets your mind off your fear. When you actually listen to another person without thinking about how what they're saying affects you, you can relax and be present with them in the moment. Some people with social anxiety have trouble making friends, and this is the primary reason: they are so worried about their own fears that they don't get to know the other person for who they are.

How to Focus on Others

If you're ready to shift your focus from yourself to others, start by clearing your mind. Take some deep breaths and let your anxious thoughts drift out of your mind. Notice the fearful thoughts, but don't dwell on them or try to reason them out. Just let them pass quietly by like clouds passing overhead on a breezy day. Clearing your mind takes practice, and you can work on it anytime you like. Whenever your mind is filled with worried or otherwise undesirable thoughts, practice letting go of those thoughts and enjoy the serenity of having a tranquil mind.

Practice Active Listening

Make it a habit to practice active listening in your everyday interactions. Active listening is a technique that allows you to hear the other person and get feedback to make sure you understand. Here's how you do it. If the other person hasn't said anything yet, ask them an open question (one that can't be answered with a simple one-word answer like yes or no). If the other person is already talking, just focus on their words, gestures and facial expressions and pay attention to what they're saying.

If you don't understand something the other person says, don't just let it pass unnoticed. Ask them a question to help them clarify their meaning. Then, when the other person finishes speaking, summarize what they've said and ask them if you understood them correctly. If they say "no," then ask them what it was that you misunderstood. The point of active listening is to let the other person express themselves in a way you can understand and to show the other person that you're interested in what they're saying.

Practice Empathy

The Greater Good Science Center describes empathy as "the ability to sense other people's emotions, coupled with the ability to imagine what someone else is thinking and feeling." Imagination is really the key to practicing empathy. You notice the visual and verbal cues the other person is expressing, practice active listening to understand their situation, and then use your imagination to gain a deeper understanding of what they think and feel about the situation.

However, having an empathetic understanding of someone doesn't help them at all unless your express your empathy. Start by making guesses about what they feel, based on your empathetic understanding. For example, you might say, "I'm guessing you feel sad about that," or "I imagine you're having some angry thoughts about that." Then, listen to how the person answers you. If you were wrong, make new guesses, even if it is to say, "I'm guessing you don't feel much like talking right now."

Once you've sharpened up your empathetic understanding of the person's problem, find out what they need in this moment. You can say, "I'm guessing you need some encouragement right now," or "I'm guessing you could use a hug." Then, offer to give them what they need if it's something you have to give. If not, offer to help them get the thing they need. Be there with them when they aren't feeling great, and they'll be more likely to interact well with you in the future.

Volunteer in Your Community

How can volunteer work help you get over your social anxiety? The answer is simple. If you concentrate on doing something you feel is important and beneficial to others, you'll spend less time thinking about how others react to you socially. You'll be more interested in doing something worthwhile than on socializing. The social interactions will be secondary to the good you are doing, so you'll be less self conscious about them.

Here's an example of how one woman used volunteering to get beyond her social anxiety.

Sherri was always nervous when she tried to talk to others. Because of this, she often felt lonely and misunderstood. One day, she saw a poster on the bulletin board at her job that interested her. The poster described volunteer opportunities in the community. Its caption read "Come be a part of our team!" The idea of being a part of something made her feel happy, so she called the number on the poster and set up an appointment to discuss how she could help.

The interviewer, wanting to recruit as many volunteers as possible, was very kind and encouraging. When Sherri mentioned that she liked to crochet, the volunteer coordinator suggested she give crochet lessons at a local women's shelter. It would give the women something constructive to do, help them occupy their minds, and possibly even give them a way to earn a few extra dollars each month.

Sherri was hesitant, but when she thought of the women who were uprooted from their homes, usually because of a violent spouse, she felt a strong desire to help them, if even in this small way. As she taught the classes, the women began to show that they accepted her and enjoyed her company. And, when she expressed empathy for them, many of them told her that no one understood how they felt before.

After that, when Sherri went into social situations, she thought first of what she could do for other people. She knew that any social fears she had were small compared to some of the things others have to go through, so she found it easier and easier to focus on what she could do to help them. She still had moments of social awkwardness, but she had learned to place less importance on those problems. She developed more social connections in her daily life than she ever had before.

When you place your focus on what someone else needs and wants, you leave less room for thoughts of your perceived social inadequacy. You are thinking of others now, so your fears are less prominent and more manageable.

Chapter 22: Tackling Anxiety

For an individual dealing with anxiety on a daily basis, it is difficult to define the agony they suffer. Extreme GAD often precludes depression and a sense of hopelessness of having to live with the worry and tension each day.

Let us go through a comprehensive list of symptoms of persons suffering from GAD:

Excessive anxiety, without a base reason for the worry

Overwhelming fear and uneasiness

Restlessness, and feeling constantly on edge

Tension in upper body muscles leading to pain in neck, shoulders and back from constant stiffness

Headaches and nausea

Loss of appetite

Breathlessness

Irritability

Trembling of extremities, such as fingers or lips

Insomnia or trouble staying asleep

Exhaustion from constantly being restless

Whilst it is known that GAD is diffused anxiety, that is anxiety without reason, there are also triggers which spur an anxiety attack. More often than not, the anxiety once triggered, lingers in a diffused state. For instance, a patient who is staying away from home may that they would never see their sister again.

Once triggered, the anxiety would linger on, and each time the individual thinks of her sister and the distance between them, the anxiety would strengthen, causing the anxiety attack to either recur or worsen.

At the same time, the anxiety would exist in a diffused state, such that the person continues to feel anxious despite not having thoughts of their sister throughout the day. This is because the thought of the patient's sister is only the trigger. It is not the main concern for the person.

Excessive anxiety can also lead to panic attacks, but as we have seen earlier, this does not mean that the individual is suffering from Panic Disorder. The panic attacks are a result of the anxiety going beyond what the individual can handle.

This is important to understand for any treatment to be effective. Anxiety Disorders are treated in mostly the same way that Panic Disorders are treated. The patient is offered the following:

- Psychotherapy as a treatment, by regular visits to the psychotherapist
- Use of modern medicine, that is, Benzos (anti-anxiety medication)

- The treatment can be enhanced with the use of both psychotherapy and Benzos
- If the patient has an advanced case of anxiety and is also suffering from depression, antidepressants may also be prescribed.

Selective Serotonin Reuptake Inhibitors (SSRIs), are a form of anti-depressants which are used to treat depression, unexplained panic attacks and anxiety. For persons suffering from chronic anxiety disorders such as GAD, citalopram (Celexa), escitalopram (Lexapro), and sertraline (Zoloft) are often prescribed.

SNRIs (serotonin and norepinephrine reuptake inhibitors) are compounds which work to either produce or suppress enzymes in the brain such as serotonin and norepinephrine. Antihistamines and beta-blockers are used in alternate cases where a person's GAD is not severe.

The condition that follows SSRIs or SNRIs is that the tablet has to be taken on a daily basis as long as it has been prescribed by the doctor, regardless of whether the individual is suffering from anxiety attacks on a particular day.

On the other hand, Antihistamines or beta-blockers are prescribed on a per need basis and are to be taken only if the patient is suffering from anxiety, or has identified a trigger for anxiety.

A drug that is prescribed to all patients with chronic anxiety is a set of drugs classified as benzodiazepines; alprazolam (Xanax) and diazepam (Valium). However, taking Benzodiazepines on a regular basis causes side effects such as memory problems, excessive drowsiness and irritability. Taking them in a large dose for a short period of time to overcome severe anxiety is, however, safe.

Whilst it is important to consult a doctor, it is also necessary that the individual tries to overcome anxiety on a personal level. We have here some techniques that are useful for fighting extreme anxiety.

Psychotherapy:

Psychotherapy, as a standalone option or in conjunction with medication, is thought to be a fundamental option of treatment for generalised anxiety disorder. The main point of psychotherapy is to 'talk your way out of anxiety'. Different Talk Therapies have different guide ways.

Out of the multiple therapies that are applied, there are several methods which have been found to be more applicable and effective than others. Psychodynamic psychotherapy and Supportive-expressive therapy are two particular therapies which allow the individual to look at anxiety differently. They prescribe to the worry being an outgrowth of fears and worries about relationships important to the person.

Here we discuss some forms of psychotherapy which are used to effectively treat GAD:

- Acceptance & Commitment Therapy – ACT is a form of 'third-wave' therapy. This is a three part therapy, which focuses on behavioural conditioning and processing in the first two waves, and follows a route of acceptance in the third wave.

ACT is, as the name suggests, an acceptance therapy, in which through talking, the sufferer is guided to accept their disorder. This follows on the theory that when you stop fighting the symptoms, you stop the constant train of thoughts running in your mind about the symptoms. This, in turn, allows for greater psychological flexibility.

Acceptance of your circumstance is designed to protect the mind from anxiety triggers and painful thoughts. As a result, the individual has turned into the patterns of their thoughts, avoidance mechanism, and actions they take. Identifying these patterns allows the sufferer to understand how and what would trigger their anxiety, and how to tackle it more efficiently.

For instance, let us look at Sue who is having triggers which cause anxiety attacks to begin. Thoughts of her mother bring on anxiety, which lasts through the day. By getting Sue to talk about her innermost fears, the psychotherapist would understand what is going on in her mind which causes her to be anxious about her mother.

By identifying what causes her mother to give her anxiety, the psychotherapist would be in a better position to lead Sue's thoughts to think positively.

It is important that to avail ACT, you need to approach a psychologist trained in this type of psychotherapy. Your psychotherapist should be empathetic and be willing to listen and hear you out. At the same, he should be non-judgemental as he guides you through your conversations exploring your anxiety, bringing about an awareness of your emotions.

In a typical session, you will practice mindfulness to look at your thoughts. This means not judging your own thoughts, instead of having a positive awareness of your emotions, memories and sensations. Once your deepest thoughts and fears are identified, the therapist would sit through cognitive exercises to redefine and put into perspective your story, to help you to accept it as what it is – just an experience of life.

- Psychodynamic Psychotherapy: Psychodynamic is based on a theory that the subconscious mind has feelings and thoughts of its own, which can lead to inner conflicts that emerge as anxiety attacks.

This would mean that Sue has worries which she is not consciously aware of, but that are present at the back of her mind, which causes her anxiety. As she is not able to pinpoint at these thoughts because they are not present in her conscious thoughts, the anxiety she feels exists in a diffused form.

By talking about her feelings, and identifying what it is that is present in her sub-conscious mind that causes her to feel anxiety about her mother, Sue would get relief from her anxiety symptoms.

During therapy, a patient is encouraged to talk freely about their feelings and emotions in an attempt to make them aware of their sub-conscious minds. This is an unstructured therapy, and not defined by a carefully crafted script, and may continue over a long period of time.

Individuals availing this therapy find it very effective in reducing anxiety symptoms. However, as the therapy takes a long time to work, and is unstructured, short-term psychodynamic therapy is emerging as a new branch.

- Interpersonal Psychotherapy: IPT was originally designed to treat depression. However, as it was found to be very effective in treating anxiety symptoms arising due to depression, it has been extended for anxiety treatment too.

IPT is a form of therapy which looks at anxiety being a manifestation of the worries and tensions which arise due to problems in relationships. This therapy believes that resolving relationship problems will resolve anxiety issues.

IPT looks at Sue's relationship with her mother as a cause of the anxiety attacks she suffers. By talking about her problems, and improving her relationship, her anxiety would also go away. By understanding the issues in her relationship, Sue's therapist would be able to pinpoint the areas which are causing the anxiety to arise, and how to deal with it.

A typical therapy session can be a personal session with the therapist, or a group therapy session where listening to other sufferers talk about their problems will help the individual identify their own issues.

These are short, concise sessions which are time-limited and focused only on the present life of the person. The patient would ideally talk about a few relationships that are particular to them, and the issues they face in those relationships. The therapy also focuses on improving communication techniques of the patient to improve the overall interpersonal effectiveness in their daily lives.

As such, for persons diagnosed with depression made severe by GAD, IPT is a very effective form of therapy that can be applied.

- Cognitive Behavioural Therapy: CBT is unlike other therapy options, in the sense it focuses on the present and conscious mind of the individual, rather than the sub-conscious. It is a form of structured problem-solving therapy.

Ideally, CBT is a short-term therapy that can be extended to a longer period if the GAD symptoms of the individual wax and wane over a long period of time. The focus of CBT is to enable the sufferer to identify their own problems, in an attempt to make them their own therapist.

This would mean that Sue is suffering from anxiety attacks related to thoughts of her mother because she has active thoughts about her mother – either related to her health, her relationship, or other causes.

By understanding what it on her mind and not avoiding those thoughts, Sue would be able to fight the anxiety symptoms more effectively.

CBT has to be taken from a therapist who is trained in it. Interesting, a therapist can be a psychiatrist, a psychologist or a mental health counsellor. A typical session would be very active, taking the patient on a journey of reflecting upon their issues through educative conversations.

CBT will guide the individual to understand their anxiety better by analysing their own selves, learning to let go and relax, and reining in their thoughts. This is done by using a variety of CBT approaches, learning to stop avoiding facing their fears, and starting to focus on a problem-solving lifestyle for the issues that may cause anxiety.

During the CBT session, the therapist will team up with the individual to agree upon the agenda for the sessions. All sessions will focus on homework, to have the patient practice the techniques that have been studied during the session. The therapist will review the homework to ensure the individual is making an effort too.

The sessions are usually carried out weekly unless the anxiety symptoms are out of control. In such cases, the sessions will be increased to support the sufferer, until the anxiety comes under control. Post the sessions, once the individual recovers from their anxiety symptoms, patients may return to visit with their therapist for 'booster' sessions, as a check-in on their self-therapy.

By talking with their doctor, individuals may identify which form of psychotherapy would be most suitable for them.

Alternately, you may understand each type of psychotherapy and decide which one you would prefer referring to help alleviate your anxiety symptoms.

To understand some basic home exercises which persons suffering from GAD may practice, let us go on to the next chapter.

Chapter 23: Speak Your Mind

People who are shy and anxious tend to have a hard time speaking what is on their minds. They do not speak up even when they feel the need to. They become afraid and hesitant. They also become fearful of gaining any unwanted attention. They are typically quiet and soft-spoken. Well, if you keep bottling up your thoughts and emotions, you might break down. Hence, it is very important for you to learn to speak up when necessary.

Voice Out Your Opinions. If you have an opinion about something, you should not be afraid to let other people know about it. For instance, if you are at a meeting and you want to suggest a new technique or method, you should speak up. Tell everyone in the meeting room about your suggestion and explain how it can benefit the company.

Do not let your good ideas be wasted just because you are shy or anxious of being rejected. If they reject your idea, then move on. Do not wallow or hold a grudge. Do not think that you are not good enough either. You should not take things personally, especially at work. It is crucial for you to learn how to view things in an objective manner rather than in a subjective one.

Likewise, if you do not agree about something, you should not hesitate to say so. You should not antagonize the person though. See to it that you express yourself in a reasonable manner. You should also be open to the suggestions and opinions of other people. If someone has a negative opinion about your suggestion, you can take that as a form of criticism to help you come up with better suggestions.

If someone attempts to undermine you by making snide remarks or rude comments, you should not go down to the level of that person. If you continue to display a good attitude at work, you can get promoted and your co-workers will admire you. Achieving good things can make you feel better about yourself and reduce your self-consciousness.

Do Not Let Other People Bully You. It is not uncommon for bullies to exist at school and the workplace. People bully their peers for various reasons. Some of them do it because they want to feel in control while others do it as a form of compensation for their own weakness. There are people who bully others because they feel threatened or insecure.

Nonetheless, no matter what the reason of the bully is, you should not allow him to torment or undermine you. Do not be afraid to defend yourself. You should speak up and tell the bully to stop. You should not fight back though. Instead, you should empathize with him and try to understand where he is coming from. This will help you determine how you can handle your situation better.

You may talk to him one on one and find out what his problem is. Talk to him and maybe even offer to help him out. He may be lashing out on you because he has problems at home. Remember that if you do nothing, there will be no change. If you want the bullying to stop, you have to do something about it. If you are able to defend yourself, people will admire your courage and give you respect.

Introduce Yourself. Due to your social anxiety, you may find it stressful to attend parties and mingle with other people. You may have a hard time dealing with acquaintances and total strangers. Because of this, you deny yourself of numerous possibilities.

Let us say that you are good at singing and you attend a big event with well-renowned guests. You spot a talent manager. Do you fight the urge to approach him for fear of being ignored or rejected or do you come up to him and introduce yourself.

If you dream of selling albums and being a famous singer, you should gather up your courage and walk up to the talent manager. Introduce yourself and start a conversation. You can ask him to listen to your demo tape or voice recording. If he declines, you can politely insist to give you a chance. You can also leave him your calling card.

For all you know, this could be your chance of achieving your dreams. Do not cut yourself short. You deserve better and you should know that. Stop being self-conscious and insecure. You have to believe that you are capable of making your dreams come true.

Learn to Say No. Some people have a hard time saying "no". They do not decline offers or requests because they fear that the other person will get mad or disappointed. They try so hard to please everybody even if it means displeasing themselves. Because of this, they end up suffering.

If you want to be happy, you should learn to say "no" once in a while. For instance, if you are exhausted from work and someone calls you to invite you to a party, do you either say "yes" and go or do you say "no" and stay home to rest?

If you go to the party, you will not be able to enjoy yourself because you are tired. You will also be late for work the next day and this will only make you more anxious.

If you politely decline the offer and explain your reasons, you will not ruin your relationship with your friend. Moreover, you will have the opportunity to rest, rejuvenate yourself, and get ready for a new day.

Waking up refreshed can keep you in a good mood all day and allow you to find more opportunities. Furthermore, not being able to say "no" will only make you a doormat. When you allow this to happen, other people will not respect you. Hence, you should learn how to put boundaries.

Chapter 24: Hard Trauma And Soft Trauma

Psychologists define a hard trauma as a stressful event which has a profound impact on the mind and or body. Examples of hard trauma would be suffering a serious injury in a motor accident or being physically attacked in your home by a stranger. Such experiences can lead to post-traumatic stress disorder, where the nervous system becomes acutely dysregulated and the sufferer can experience frightening flashbacks and dramatic mood swings in response to minor stresses. However, many psychologists now believe that chronic soft trauma can also be very distressing and disabling. A soft trauma is a moderately stressful event that the rational mind doesn't consider particularly stressful but which is experienced as traumatic by the person involved. For example, most people would not consider going to a lively party very stressful, but someone with a high level of social anxiety might be somewhat traumatised by the experience. Similarly, watching a horror film isn't likely to be a very stressful experience for most adults but it could well be traumatic for an impressionable child. So any mild to moderately stressful situation can be experienced as traumatic if the person experiencing it feels helpless and doesn't have the capacity to be able to cope with the (real or imagined) threat. The accumulative effects of trauma can be particularly problematic for individuals with ongoing life problems that can't be easily resolved. For example, people with learning disabilities that start in childhood may experience a lot of soft trauma while growing up and may subsequently develop very dysregulated autonomic nervous systems.*

*Numerous studies indicate that people with learning disorders, ADHD, speech problems such as stuttering, gender dysphoria, and chronic painful conditions such as fibromyalgia and arthritis have above average rates of anxiety and depression.

Social Anxiety

Among the various sub-types of mood disorders, social anxiety is arguably the one that is most directly influenced by personal trauma. Social anxiety affects at least seven percent of the population and is equally common in males and females. It is most common in teenagers and young adults and is less common in older adults. It's likely that some people who experience significant social anxiety have an in-born predisposition towards experiencing negative emotions. However, the vast majority of people with social anxiety also have a history of soft or hard trauma that makes them overly sensitive to social judgment by others. Such trauma can include bullying by school mates or older siblings, excessive criticism by parents, unpleasant interactions with strangers, or negative experiences with authority figures. Because social anxiety is heavily influenced by past trauma it tends to respond very well to brain-body therapies that help to discharge physical tension and dissipate traumatic memories. In particular, tension release exercises can be very effective in helping people with social anxiety feel less self-conscious and more at ease in social situations.

Dissociation

Mild to moderate dissociation is a relatively common defensive reaction to stressful or traumatic events and is relatively common in people suffering from anxiety and depression. Dissociation is a disruption in the normally integrated functions of memory, consciousness, and awareness of the outside world. It can also interfere with a person's sense of identity and leave them feeling like they are a spectator in their own lives. Symptoms of dissociation can range from simple lapses of attention, such as everyday forgetfulness, to depersonalisation and loss of memory for important events. In some respects, chronic, moderate dissociation is a less extreme but more chronic version of the freeze response observed in the animal world. * In the freeze response, endorphins are released by the nervous system so there is a numbing of physical feelings and an altered state of consciousness. This helps us to stay physically calm and protects us from unnecessary mental and physical pain in the event of being physically attacked by a predator. In modern humans, mild to moderate dissociation helps to preserve our mental stability and reduce stress-related physical illness by shielding us from painful memories and experiences that we don't have the capacity to deal with.

*Psychologist Stephen Porges points out that medical researchers have known about many of the physical and mental effects of the fight and flight responses for over a century, but it is only in the last few decades that they have started to appreciate the mental and physical effects of the freeze response.

According to trauma researcher Pete Walker, people with dysregulated nervous systems from trauma tend to fall into certain types, based on certain factors such as in-born temperament and family upbringing. These dysregulated types coincide with the flight, fight and freeze responses found in nature. People with relatively passive personalities tend to favour the freeze response and are therefore more prone to dissociation. Characteristics of the chronic freeze response include: dissociation, social isolation, daydreaming, inattention, couch potato behaviour, and fear of success. Walker argues that freeze types tend to avoid relationships and hide their personal feelings. They also tend to avoid face to face encounters with strangers as they subconsciously associate strangers with danger.

Dissociation versus Attention Deficit Disorder

In the mental health field, the line between what is considered inattention and what is considered dissociation is pretty fuzzy. Most psychologists would consider missing parts of a conversation due to day dreaming as inattention, whereas not recognising friends or blanking out significant events would be considered pathological dissociation. The general view at present is there is a moderate degree of overlap between ADD symptoms and dissociative symptoms, and this overlap is consistent for both genders. Certainly both ADD and dissociation can occur in early childhood and continue to produce significant attentional problems in adulthood. Subsequently, anyone diagnosed with either ADD or dissociation should be screened for both disorders. In cases where inattention is primarily caused by dissociation, it is unlikely that the person in question will benefit from ADD medications like Adderall as these will tend to increase over-arousal of the sympathetic nervous system and may actually worsen their tendency to dissociate. Symptoms of dissociation also tend to be more common in those with ADD without hyperactivity, and individuals with this form of ADD are more likely to experience anxiety and depression, and are less likely to respond favourably to commonly prescribed stimulant medications.

Chapter 25: **You Have The Power**

In conclusion, you have the power to create the environment you want. You are 10% of what happens to you and 90% of how you react to it.

When you are faced with a situation, do not worry, do not panic, just seek understanding. DO not be ignorant. The wisest man to have ever walked the face of the earth once said, "in all your seeking, seek understanding." So all in all, it's not what happens to you, but how you react to it that matters.

There are two sides, always stick to the **right one**.

Negative side (-)	Positive side (+)
1. Exposed to information	1.Exposed to information
2. Ignorance	2.Knowledge
3. Negative ideas/thoughts	3.Understanding
4. Fear	4.Faith

5. Anxiety	5. Well-being
6. Depression	6. Confidence
7. Dis-ease	7. At-ease
8. Disintergration	8. Creation

It is worth mentioning that you acquire knowledge and understanding through studying, asking questions from people with experience and taking the necessary action.

ABOUT THE AUTHOR

After obtaining my Bachelor of Commerce Degree, I was very eager to go out there and make a difference in the real world of business. I started working as a call center agent in one of the most prestigious mobile operators that I will not mention for ethical reasons. Within a few months I moved to another company (a bank) where I worked as a bank teller.

My job was fine, the salary was fair, but I was not happy, I wanted to be financially free, I didn't want to work in an 8 to 5 job anymore, practically I wanted to be my own boss. I was sick and tired of asking for permissions, scheduling my vacations at times convenient to the bank, worrying about meeting the needs and obligations of my family, working on Saturdays, student and personal loans.

I made a decision to change my life, but I had no idea where to start, I tried attending some success seminars, I tried the law of attraction, I tried meditation, visualization, I tried the lottery, I tried online trading, but nothing seemed to work.

The turning point of my life

In the summer of 2015 everything changed, the bank had a habit of inviting its top (premium) clients to dine with the executive and some members of staff, just as a way of appreciating them and acknowledging their support. Luckily enough for me, I was part of the few lower staff invited to be part of the occasion.

Everyone was allowed to meet and chat with all of the top clients during the refreshments hour, it was more like a socializing event. In the nick of time I saw an opportunity to push my own agenda, after all I wanted to be rich, and there I was in the room with the richest people in the city.

As a bank teller I knew all their bank accounts statuses and balances but I couldn't discuss this with just any one since the bank had all employees sign NDA's (non-disclosure agreements) which made it a crime to discuss client's accounts with third parties.

So I decided to grab the opportunity and went to have a chat with each of the clients, I thanked them for banking with Us, admired their success, asked what line of business they were in and if they had any advice for a young chap like me, on how to be successful and be like them some day.

Of course as you can imagine they just laughed when they heard this. But most of these top guns were eager to throw in some advice whilst some were reserved and protective, they just did not want to mention how they made their wealth or how someone else could do it.

One of the top clients was Mr. Sam ChaMichel (God bless his soul) an 83 years old man who was the town's real estate mogul, business magnate and leading philanthropist. Most people in the city referred to him as Sam the Tycoon or just Old Sam.

At the time his bank account had Millions of dollars, taking this money into consideration, his successful real estate investments and the couple of other businesses he owned, it was just clear to me that this man was very successful a true Millionaire that I wanted to idolize.

I was really hesitant about going to Mr. Sam, he didn't look like the kind that tolerated small talk, I decided to take my chances. I went over to start a conversation with him. After answering a couple of his questions, I threw in mine, and to my surprise Old Sam did not only answer my questions with enthusiasm, but he gave me a brief lecture on the basics of success.

To summarize, Mr. Sam taught me the following concepts:

... Knowledge is only potential power. True power is the application of knowledge.

….There is a huge difference between preparing to kill a lion and actually killing the lion.

... Data on its own can't help you, instead it will only confuse you, but if that data is processed, organized, structured and interpreted, it becomes meaningful and useful.

At the end of our conversation, after all we didn't have enough time, he said with a slight grin;

"Boy judging from your questions, you have all of the data needed in order to become successful, but that data is useless and meaningless on its own, you need someone to help you organize, arrange, interpret, and show you how to use it, and that's where I come in.

After 4 months, of Mr. Sam's lessons, I started a small business and I worked on it during my spare time. Using Mr. Sam's concepts, I expanded the business and I started focusing more on expanding my customer base. 6 months later when my net income from my business was equal to my salary from the bank, I left the bank and I totally focused on my business.

I now own 2 very productive companies, I no longer work full time in any of them. My monthly income now greatly exceeds my monthly expenses, making me financially independent. I made my **First 1 Million Dollars** exactly 2 years after quitting my job at the bank, and if you are interested on the other things Mr. Sam taught me, kindly send me an email at: vincentking340@gmail.com and it will be my privilege to share with you the blue print to real wealth.

Chapter 26: Supplements

Here are some supplements that you can take to ease your Social Anxiety:

L-Tyrosine: This is a supplement that has been known to help to treat anxiety of all kinds. Tyrosine is an amino acid that has been found to be useful during conditions of stress, cold, fatigue, but has not been found to have any significant effect on mood, cognitive or physical performance in normal circumstances.

L-theanine: Theanine is an amino acid commonly found in tea, and also in the basidiomycete mushroom Boletus badius. Theanine is related to glutamine, and can cross the blood-brain barrier .Because it can enter the brain, theanine has psychoactive properties. Theanine has been shown to reduce mental and physical stress, may produce feelings of relaxation and improves cognition and mood when taken in combination with caffeine.

Chamomile: Those from North America are probably most familiar with chamomile in the form of tea. Often we drink chamomile tea before bed for the calming and sedating effects that it is supposed to induce. Surprisingly, however, not enough scientific research has been conducted to support the anti-anxiety properties of this herbal supplement. However, if you find drinking a cup of chamomile tea tends to calm your nerves before a social engagement that may be all the evidence you need.

Winter Cherry (ashwagandha): Winter cherry (withania somnifera), also known as ashwagandha or Indian ginseng, has traditionally been used as part of a holistic system of medicine in India known as Ayurveda. The herbal supplement is produced from the root of the plant and is known as an adaptogen, meaning that it increases resistance to physical and emotional stress. In terms of emotional health, winter cherry has been used to promote emotional balance in cases of mild anxiety, depression and mental or physical fatigue. The supplement is also known to have many preventative qualities, such as anti-inflammatory and antioxidant properties.

Phenibut: Beta-phenyl-gamma-amino butyric acid, better known as Phenibut or less commonly Fenibut or Phenybut, is natural derivative of the inhibitory neurotransmitter GABA (Gamma amino butyric acid). Sold as a dietary supplement in the US while in Russia sold as a neuropsychotropic drug that is capable of passing the blood-brain barrier. Phenibut is cited as a nootropic for its ability to improve neurological functions. It was discovered in Russia in the 1960's, and has since been used there to treat a wide range of ailments including anxiety and insomnia.

Here are some medicines that you can take if you have a serious condition and are seeking medical attention as a last resort, I am in no way responsible for your choice to take these drugs and by doing so, you are at your own risk. Also, consult a doctor before taking any supplements/ Drugs.

Paroxitine (Paxil). This is an anti-depressant drug which is orally administered. This is used to treat panic attacks, insomnia, aggressive or hostile behavior, and aids in the dissolution of suicidal or self-harmful thoughts.

Fluoxetine (Prozac, Sarafem, others). These are types of Uppers that are used in the treatment of Bulimia Nervosa, Depression, Panic Attacks, and Premenstrual Dysphoric Disorder.

Sertraline (Zoloft).This is one of those Serotonin Reuptake Inhibitors, more commonly known as Uppers. Serotonin is the part of the brain that is responsible for feelings of happiness and that's why people with low Serotonin levels are most commonly depressed. By taking this drug, you can be able to feel better and lighter and get more happy hormones.

Fluvoxamine (Luvox). This is a drug used for treating several psychiatric disorders. It is also a kind of Upper that gives you more happy hormones and increases your Serotonin level. It has also been approved as a medicine for those with Obsessive-Compulsive Disorders.

Clonazepam (Kloponin). A drug which is best used for phobias, generalized anxiety and social anxiety.

Beta Blockers such as Propanolol and Atenolol. These are best for social anxiety. These are also the most recommended types of drugs for those who have Social Anxieties as they have been used for years and have been tried and tested by many.

Tricyclic Anti-Depressants such as Imipramine, Despiramine, Doxepin, and Clomipramine. These are best in the treatment of Post-Traumatic Stress

Disorders, Social Anxiety, Obsessive-Compulsive Disorders, Panic Attacks and Depression.

Buspirone. This is a tranquilizer that stabilizes someone who has anxieties, panic attacks and Obsessive-Compulsive Disorders.

Venlafaxine. This is recommended for those who have sever social anxieties.

Some people with Social Anxiety Disorder recommend the use of energy drinks such as Red Bull or the use of herbal medicines such as St. John's Wort before going out and engaging in social situations as these increase energy and can make someone feel better which is important from those suffering from Social Anxiety.

Remember to consult with a doctor first before taking in any medicines and please do not take all these medicines all together. Especially if you haven't checked with a physician first. It's never good to self-medicate especially in cases like this.

This is just a guide as to what you can take when you feel like you have Social Anxiety.

Chapter 27: The Ultimate Cheat Sheet On

Introverts At Work

As an introvert, or someone who works with Introverts, there are always things you can learn that will help you work more effectively with one another. It doesn't mean you aren't all working together famously right now; it means to think how fantastic it could be if you could all "up" your game. Think of this like the owner's manual to your car. Sure, you can drive it but are you really taking advantage of all the features you bought?

Let's set the stage for the fundamental personality differentiator: energy.

Introverts develop maintain and restore their energy by what goes on in their head. It's the "inner" world. When being at a party or meetings exhausts them, they immediately seek solitude. The solitude allows them to restore their energy. It can also be the thing that causes them to be quiet in a meeting. Think of it like autopilot. Their autopilot is maintaining their energy by listening rather than talking.

The other thing about Introverts is that when they speak, it's for a reason or purpose. They aren't prone to "thinking out-loud." Now, there's your quick lesson. Let's apply this to how that shows up in the workplace.

- They may need time to think. If you pop something on them, don't always expect a quick answer.

- They aren't being anti-social when they stay in their office. They're doing what they do best - hunker down, focus and think. In fact, they would welcome you to provide a break but just don't expect to see them until the work is done.

- They will give talks or presentations. Just because they don't speak up in a meeting, doesn't mean they won't gladly prepare something to share with the group. This situation means they have a purpose to speak - it makes so much sense now doesn't it?

- They make relationships and therefore influence one-on-one. Don't expect to see the introvert get all "over-the-top" about something in order to persuade or influence others. On the other hand, don't make the mistake of thinking they don't have tons of influence because those relationships are deep and tight - just the right mix for tremendous influence.

- They will be fairly quiet in meetings. This is because they are listening and in their energy conservation mode. However, if you need to have them contributing to discussions either ask them specifically their opinion or ask ahead of time to contribute in the meeting.

- They tend to not be too self-promoting. If you can help in this area, do so. Introverts, like everyone else, have a wealth of capability to offer and they don't always really let their light shine. This may hamper their career growth and become a source of unhappiness. For the management of this person, they may not really be deploying a good asset.

- They can do everything an extrovert can do. A myth in our culture is that introverts don't work in sales, marketing, business ownership or even acting. Talk about stereotyping. You will find them in all occupations. They may not do the work the same way an extrovert might, but they get the job done. And, that's what matters, right?

As an introvert, you may need to make some momentary adjustments to your style to suit the situation. As a person who works with an introvert, a well-placed question or request is all it takes to unleash their power.

Chapter 28: Mind-Reading And Assuming

"To enjoy good health, to bring true happiness to one's family, to bring peace to all, one must first discipline and control one's own mind. If a man can control his mind he can find the way to Enlightenment, and all wisdom and virtue will naturally come to him."

Buddha

Mind-reading and assuming are two negative thinking processes that can manipulate your mind and can cause social anxiety problems. No matter how hard you try or how smart you are, you will never be able to read the minds of other people.

Many people believe that they know what other people are thinking based on the look on the person's face or how they act towards them. These biased assumptions and rendering in your brain can hinder your journey towards happiness.

For example, throughout different types of scenarios, phrases like "he is angry at me", "are they saying bad things about me?", "they are going to hate me" are all typical patterns for people to show when they are trying to mindread. They are assuming the worst.

The truth is you will never know what a person is really thinking about unless you directly ask them for their thoughts on that specific topic. Try to be aware when you are thinking about these things such as uncertainties, negative questioning, fears, anxieties, or a negative issue that needs clarification. Try not to repress your pain or worry about how the other person is thinking, but instead turn it into a positive. You might want to consider the possibility that people are not even speaking or thinking bad things about you, instead, you should convince yourself that they are speaking good things about you. For example, if you see someone that is looking at you a bit strangely, think to yourself that they're looking at how unique and special you are. Try to trick your brain into focusing more on the positive side of situations by accepting it as a fact. People are only thinking good things about you, and if they are in reality thinking bad things, you should not concern yourself with it, as it is negative, you should simply accept it as an issue that the other person has to resolve within themselves, maybe that other person is chronically a negative person and should read this book.

Stay truthful to yourself, think positively about yourself, and whatever the case, do not let others influence your thoughts.

The belief that you can read minds is false, you never know what other people are thinking. Mind reading is a form of miscommunication where negative thoughts jump into your mind without you consciously putting them there. Most of the time we believe that these negative thoughts are true because it is very strong and has too much power over us. Thinking that these things are true may make us feel negative feelings such as worthlessness, judged, mistreated, or not good enough. Disarm it and take away it's power.

How to Limit Mind-Reading

We worry a lot about what other people think, and worry is also a natural negative reaction that our minds have built. Until you know for 100% fact that they do think negatively about you, as a response, you should accept it as truth that people are thinking great things about you. To trick your mind, be a little bit stubborn as you see some people who, no matter what people say to or about them, the negativity they have no control over doesn't phase them one bit; be strong! Not everyone you meet will like you, no matter how much you try, but if you build up your confidence this way, you will not care about that. Remember that you are only interested in the people that will make you feel good, empowered and positive; and the more positive you are, the fewer people will have a reason to dislike you.

Here are more tips for you to stop mind-reading other people:

- Recognize When You Are Mind Reading. If you are a frequent mind reader, pay attention to what you are thinking and try to notice whenever you are lost in thought and potentially trying to find out what other people are thinking. Once you caught yourself, consciously think about flipping it to a positive. You can also imagine that thought being put in a box and thrown into outer space so that you never see it again. This is a little NLP trick that with repetition can be very powerful for the way your mind works. We'll discuss NLP in another chapter.
- Worst Case Scenario: Think to yourself how realistic are these thoughts you're projecting upon other people? Do you think that everybody is always thinking

about you? In all fairness, probably not. Even if they do, what is the possible worst case of scenario? It's really not that bad...

- Accept Yourself. The main reason we mind read other people is that we feel afraid that other people are talking about our insecurities. In all reality, we cannot stop people from talking about us. What you must do is learn how to accept and how to love yourself because you're the only person that you really need to understand

Chapter 29: Understanding Where Your Shyness And Anxieties Are Coming From

Humans are inherently social beings. We seek the company of others as a response to the instinctive biological need for connection. Being in the company of other people is an evolutionary mechanism designed to increase our chances of survival, as opposed to going at it alone, which leaves us to deal with various threats on our own, thereby reducing our chances for survival in the process.

But this need to be with other people is not at all a simple thing. In fact, the very nature of human interaction is marked by a complex layer of emotions and motivations, including shyness.

Shyness is an emotion that exhibits itself in the form of social withdrawal and a desire to not get involved in social situations. In certain respects, it is the product of one's insecurities and fears. For example, when you suffer from anxiety as a result of the fact that you need to speak before an audience, you are affirming your fear of humiliating yourself in public or fear of committing a blunder and being the subject of ridicule by others.

Totally normal behavior

Experts on social behavior say that shyness is a naturally occurring emotion that reaches its peak during the adolescence stage or those awkward teenage years. Remember those? This is the period when you undergo various chemical and physical changes on your body, so you are essentially left to deal with a variety of conflicting thoughts and emotions. As a result, you tend to be more reclusive and your tendencies to become withdrawn are highlighted, too.

Shyness during this critical period is seen as a crucial element that is meant to help you overcome the various challenges along the way by strengthening your social and emotional skills. The more you are able to successfully deal with your shyness, the more adept you become at handling social situations and the more stable your character becomes.

Shyness can also be an outcome of your genetic makeup. This is precisely the reason why some people seem to be more predisposed to experience shyness than others. Experts believe that genetic attributes derived from the genes of both parents can have a lasting impact on the lives of their children, particularly if the parents themselves exhibited manifestations of shyness. While there may be a predisposition or set point for social shyness, please understand that you are not predestined to a life of unfulfilling social interactions. Like any starting point, with deliberate practice any skill can be improved.

Quality of environment

While genetics may create a set point or starting line, shyness also has an environmental component to it. In other words, it is influenced in large part by the kind of social environment and experiences you had growing up.

For instance, the kind of environment you have with your family can be a telling signal of whether you will grow up shy or not. Kids who weren't exposed to various social situations or who were not given the chance to develop their social skills in a safe environment are more likely to grow up with stunted social skills than those kids who were given the opportunity to grow these skills early on in life successfully.

An overprotective household can also play a key role in the way someone deals with shyness. Kids in an overprotective environment usually are under high scrutiny with every move carefully observed. There can be judgment and punishment leading to behaviors that are out of line which contribute to anxiety and a fear of making a wrong move.

Similarly, a high-pressure environment that does not leave any room for mistakes can breed insecurity. This is because such an environment puts an immense pressure on you to succeed, often at the expense of everything else. Because of this mindset, nothing is worse than experiencing failure. This fear of failing, coupled with the fear of disappointing others, can only result in two things: you either become obsessed at achieving success or you develop an aversion to being around other people as a way of reducing the pressure on yourself.

A cursory look at shyness as a normal human emotion may show that for the most part it is harmless. However, when left unchecked or when you are unable to handle it properly, shyness can also be a debilitating condition. The succeeding chapter discusses in detail the negative impact of shyness on your personal, social, and professional life.

Chapter 30: Today Is A New Day

Today is a new day and lots of people don't remember that. I always wake up in the morning and think it's a new beginning and I can do anything I want if I choose too. I think we all take life for granted and we get into slumps and we don't appreciate everything around us. Most people hold onto their past and don't have the courage to let it go and one of the reasons is that's where they have learnt everything that they know now. I know you have had times in your past where you have felt happy, confident and excited about certain things but you choose to focus on everything negative in your life instead of the positive. We all do it and we give major significance to small problems and it controls our entire thinking.

People that complain about their problems to me put me in a position where I can either go down to their level and say one day you'll feel better or I can tell them the harsh reality. One of my top values is honestly and I will never lie to someone to make them feel better because I have seen so many people that just have no willpower to change or have no back bone to move forward in their life. When I work with people one of the biggest obstacles in them is talking about their ugly past and this happened to them in their past.

I know people personally that have been traumatised by their past but they decided to give it a different meaning which is very inspiring to me. I have no sympathy for people that BS themselves with stories because I know if you want to get back on your feet I can't do it for you. At the end of your life your either going to have regret or you're going to be proud because you lived life to the fullest. Ever since I decided to turn my life around when I was younger I decided to make it my mission in life just to live my life to the fullest and stop living in this pity pot of excuses. People tell me all the time I don't have the looks, money, education or the family support to do what I want to do. You need to understand an excuse is just noise that comes out of your mouth that gives you nothing but certainty.

Most people I talk to in normal conversations tell me a bunch of excuses that just simply keep them stuck in their own walls of life and it keeps them safe. A safe life is not going to be a very fulfilled life and if you can understand that it should motivate you to take action. This is the one secret that I give people that are in a rut of thinking and need a way to start moving forward. I tell them to do something dangerous meaning do something you would never usually do to shock your nervous system. I said in the first chapter that whatever Identity that you have right now is keeping you trapped so you need to start doing things that you aren't used to. I want you to be loud, be number one and just focus on making progress.

Now if I'm talking to the person that doesn't know what to do you need to start trusting yourself more. Most people want to get told exactly what to do but this is your life, you need to trust yourself and ask yourself, what could I do right now that would be a little crazy but would give me a rush. Your biggest problem right now would get neurologically changed if you stepped up right now and started challenging yourself. Will you be scared at times through this process? Yes. Will you have to handle your emotions throughout this journey? Yes. One big distinction I learnt off one of my mentors was whatever traumatises you in the moment will make you expand and grow and you will grow self esteem from doing so. Everyone asks me the question how do I get over low self esteem and the answer is doing what you're afraid of.

Seriously how bad can it be and haven't you done something before and you were scared and you did it and you wanted to do it again. It's the same with everything in life it's just that anxious feeling we feel and it's either you keep it or you take action. The cure to all your fears is taking action but most people are afraid of getting rejected because they have the illusion of losing love. I remember when I kept procrastinating to take action on certain areas of my life and I would always psych myself up knowing the opportunity was right in front of me, but I would pull away. It makes you feel hopeless and worthless inside because you are about to break out to a new paradigm.

I even knew all of the stuff that I'm telling you all the techniques to make myself feel strong but I didn't have that willpower muscles built up. The front part of our brain is called the prefrontal cortex. It gets strengthen by doing things you don't want to do but making yourself fight through the pain. People that are insecure and have extreme anxiety have a weak prefrontal cortex and by challenging yourself everyday this will grow stronger and what you used to think was hard to do will get easy. So I would set up a plan for the next month to test yourself once a day to really make that front part of your brain the strongest it can be. I did a test when I was struggling and it was one of the most exhilarating months of my life and when I look back on it now it was a defining moment in my life.

This is all about you becoming a newer version of you starting today and shifting the parts of you that need to change so you can move forward. I want you to go out today and have a real life experience of controlling your emotion because reading about it won't change your life; it's all about experiencing your life. I want you to go out and fail and realize that what you're afraid off is a BS story that you are telling yourself and you will learn new distinctions that will help you in the long run. There is nothing anyone can tell you that is more powerful than doing the thing you're afraid to do.

I can show you all these new meditative tricks that will make you feel bliss for the rest of your life but I feel I would be giving you a disservice. Meditation and learning ways to relax yourself are very powerful techniques but your life will not change significantly unless you're willing to challenge and step into uncertainty. It kind of sounds extreme because I'm asking you to feel more anxious about doing this thing that scare you but all my goal for you is for you to be in control of your emotions. I will show you techniques in the following chapters that will help you manage and control your emotions but you need to be testing your limits to see the change.

I remember when I was 23 years old my mentor told me to take a chance on faith throughout your life. He told me that we have two choices in life love or fear and whichever one we choose is going to shape our destiny. He asked me what my biggest fear was. I told him not truly living my life and he said that you need to let go off all your baggage and start fresh like new were born today. Whatever happened to you in your past or the paradigm your currently living at, you have to let that go. Whether you get rejected today or you have a bad day you can always go to sleep and wake up in the morning and start fresh again today. If you can realize that you past is meant to be a learning experience and today is meant to be your life.

Most people think that if they fail in the past they are guarantee to fail in the future and of course if they go into the future using a rear view mirror of course they will crash. Realize that whatever kind of bad day you have, you can press the restart button at any time you want. I start my day fresh every single day and have a positive expectancy that maybe today I am going to do something that is going to change my life forever. There are moments in our life that change us and if you keep realizing you're in your own game of life, one action you do can change your life forever. If you fail so what, laugh about it and wake up to a new fresh day of opportunities and take advantage of every one of them.

Chapter 31: Clonazepam Pronounced As

(Kloe Na' Ze Pam)

IMPORTANT WARNING:

Clonazepam may increase the risk of serious or life-threatening breathing problems, sedation, or coma if used along with certain medications. Tell your doctor if you are taking or plan to take certain opiate medications for cough such as codeine (in Triacin-C, in Tuzistra XR) or hydrocodone (in Anexsia, in Norco, in Zyfrel) or for pain such as codeine (in Fiorinal), fentanyl (Actiq, Duragesic, Subsys, others), hydromorphone (Dilaudid, Exalgo), meperidine (Demerol), methadone (Dolophine, Methadose), morphine (Astramorph, Duramorph PF, Kadian), oxycodone (in Oxycet, in Percocet, in Roxicet, others), and tramadol (Conzip, Ultram, in Ultracet). Your doctor may need to change the dosages of your medications and will monitor you carefully. If you take clonazepam with any of these medications and you develop any of the following symptoms, call your doctor immediately or seek emergency medical care immediately: unusual dizziness, lightheadedness, extreme sleepiness, slowed or difficult breathing, or unresponsiveness. Be sure that your caregiver or family members know which symptoms may be serious so they can call the doctor or emergency medical care if you are unable to seek treatment on your own.

Drinking alcohol or using street drugs during your treatment with clonazepam also increases the risk that you will experience these serious, life-threatening side effects. Do not drink alcohol or use street drugs during your treatment.

Why is this medication prescribed?

Clonazepam is used alone or in combination with other medications to control certain types of seizures. It is also used to relieve panic attacks (sudden, unexpected attacks of extreme fear and worry about these attacks). Clonazepam is in a class of medications called benzodiazepines. It works by decreasing abnormal electrical activity in the brain.

How should this medicine be used?

Clonazepam comes as a tablet and an orally disintegrating tablet (tablet that dissolves quickly in the mouth) to take by mouth. It usually is taken one to three times a day with or without food. Take clonazepam at around the same time(s) every day. Follow the directions on your prescription label carefully, and ask your doctor or pharmacist to explain any part you do not understand.

Do not try to push the orally disintegrating tablet through the foil. Instead, use dry hands to peel back the foil packaging. Immediately take out the tablet and place it in your mouth. The tablet will quickly dissolve and can be swallowed with or without liquid.

Your doctor will probably start you on a low dose of clonazepam and gradually increase your dose, not more often than once every 3 days.

Clonazepam can be habit-forming. Do not take a larger dose, take it more often, or take it for a longer period of time or in a different way than prescribed by your doctor. Take clonazepam exactly as directed. Do not take more or less of it or take it more often than prescribed by your doctor.

Clonazepam may help control your condition, but will not cure it. It may take a few weeks or longer before you feel the full benefit of clonazepam. Continue to take clonazepam even if you feel well. Do not stop taking clonazepam without talking to your doctor, even if you experience side effects such as unusual changes in behavior or mood, If you suddenly stop taking clonazepam, you may experience withdrawal symptoms such as new or worsening seizures, hallucinating (seeing things or hearing voices that do not exist), changes in behavior, sweating, uncontrollable shaking of a part of your body, stomach or muscle cramps, anxiety, or difficulty falling asleep or staying asleep. Your doctor will probably decrease your dose gradually.

Other uses for this medicine

Clonazepam is also used to treat symptoms of akathisia (restlessness and a need for constant movement) that may occur as a side effect of treatment with antipsychotic medications (medications for mental illness) and to treat acute catatonic reactions (state in which a person does not move or speak at all or moves or speaks abnormally). Talk to your doctor about the possible risks of using this medication for your condition.

This medication is sometimes prescribed for other uses; ask your doctor or pharmacist for more information.

What special precautions should I follow?
Before taking clonazepam,

tell your doctor and pharmacist if you are allergic to clonazepam, other benzodiazepines such as alprazolam (Xanax), chlordiazepoxide (Librium, in Librax), clorazepate (Gen-Xene, Tranxene), diazepam (Diastat, Valium), estazolam, flurazepam, lorazepam (Ativan), midazolam (Versed), oxazepam, temazepam (Restoril), triazolam (Halcion), any other medications, or any of the ingredients in clonazepam tablets. Ask your pharmacist for a list of the ingredients.

tell your doctor and pharmacist what other prescription and nonprescription medications, vitamins, and nutritional supplements you are taking or plan to take. Be sure to mention any of the following: amiodarone (Cordarone, Nexterone, Pacerone); certain antibiotics such as clarithromycin (Biaxin, in Prevpac), erythromycin (Erythrocin, E-mycin, others), and troleandomycin (TAO) (not available in the US); antidepressants; certain antifungal medications such as itraconazole (Onmel. Sporanox) and ketoconazole (Nizoral); antihistamines; certain calcium channel blockers such as diltiazem (Cardizem, Tiazac, others) and verapamil (Calan, Covera, Verelan, in Tarka); cimetidine (Tagamet); HIV protease inhibitors including indinavir (Crixivan), nelfinavir (Viracept), and ritonavir (Norvir, in Kaletra); medications for anxiety, colds or allergies, or mental illness; other medications for seizures such as carbamazepine (Epitol, Tegretol, Teril), phenobarbital, phenytoin (Dilantin, Phenytek), or valproic acid (Depakene); muscle relaxants; nefazodone; rifampin (Rifadin, Rimactane); sedatives; certain selective serotonin reuptake inhibitors (SSRIs) such as fluvoxamine (Luvox); other sleeping pills; and tranquilizers. Your doctor may need to change the doses of your medications or monitor you carefully for side effects.

tell your doctor what herbal products you are taking, especially St. John's wort.

Conclusion

Thank you again for downloading this book!

Remember that being diagnosed with bipolar disorder does not mean that you have to deal with its symptoms your entire life. Yes, it can be difficult to deal with the extreme mood swings, and yes, you cannot get rid of your bipolar disorder for good, but that does not mean you can no longer live a normal and fulfilling life.

Plenty of people just like you have learned how to deal with their bipolar symptoms, and a lot of them are now able to control their episodes, or at least keep them to a bare minimum such that they are hardly noticeable. If other people can do it, so can you!

Hopefully, you were able to learn all that you need to know about bipolar disorder from this book, and with your new found knowledge, do your best to take the reins of your life and hold them tightly in your hands. Now you do not have to be a slave to your own, seemingly uncontrollable emotions; you now have the power to live your life the way you want to and not just take a back seat to your own feelings.

Finally, if you enjoyed this book, please take the time to share your thoughts and post a review on Amazon. It'd be greatly appreciated!

Thank you and good luck!

Lightning Source UK Ltd.
Milton Keynes UK
UKHW050942210822
407545UK00011B/795